The Effective Management of Post-Operative Nausea and Vomiting

Other titles in the UK Key Advances in Clinical Practice Series

The Effective Management of Breast Cancer

The Effective Management of Cancer Pain

The Effective Management of Headache

The Effective Management of Metastatic Colorectal Cancer

The Effective Management of Ovarian Cancer

The Effective Management of Benign Prostatic Disease and Lower Urinary Tract Symptoms

The Effective Management of Post-Operative Nausea and Vomiting

Edited by

Leo Strunin MD FRCA FRCPC
President of the Royal College of Anaesthetists, London, UK

David J Rowbotham MD MRCP FRCA
Professor of Anaesthesia & Pain Management, Leicester Royal Infirmary, Leicester, UK

Andrew Miles MSc MPhil PhD
UEL Professor of Health Services Research & UK Key Advances Series Organiser at St Bartholomew's Hospital, London, UK

UEL University Centre for Health Services Research

AESCULAPIUS MEDICAL PRESS
LONDON SAN FRANCISCO SYDNEY

Royal College of Anaesthetists

Published by

Aesculapius Medical Press (London, San Francisco, Sydney)
UEL University Centre for Health Services Research
St Bartholomew's Hospital
London
EC1A 7BE

First published 1999

British Library Cataloguing in Publication Data
A catalogue record for this book is available from the British Library

ISBN 1 903044 01 4

Further copies of this volume are available from:

Claudio Melchiorri
Research Dissemination Fellow
UEL Centre for Health Services Research
St Bartholomew's Hospital
London EC1 7BE

Fax: 0171 601 7085
e-mail: c.melchiorri@mds.qmw.ac.uk

Typeset, printed and bound in Britain by
Peter Powell Origination & Print Limited

Contents

Contributors

Paul LR Andrews BSc PhD, Reader in Physiology, Department of Physiology, St George's Hospital Medical School, London

Jennifer I Benton FRCA, Department of Anaesthesia, Derriford Hospital, Plymouth

Fiona Dobson MSc DipN RGN RTN, Acute Pain Nurse Specialist, University Hospital, Queen's Medical Centre, Nottingham

Steve Haigh MSc MRPharmS, Senior Pharmacist – Drug Information, King's Mill Centre for Healthcare Services NHS Trust, Sutton-in-Ashfield

Michael Harmer MD FRCA, Professor and Head of Department, Department of Anaesthetics and Intensive Care Medicine, University of Wales College of Medicine, Cardiff

Greg Hobbs BMBS FRCA, Senior Lecturer in Anaesthesia, University Department of Anaesthesia and Intensive Care, University Hospital, Queen's Medical Centre, Nottingham

Phil M Hopkins MD MB BS FRCA, Senior Lecturer in Anaesthesia, St James's University Hospital, Leeds

Philip Howard BPharm MRPharmS, Assistant Director of Pharmacy, Leeds General Infirmary, Leeds

David J Rowbotham MB ChB MD MRCP FRCA, Professor of Anaesthesia & Pain Management, University of Leicester, Leicester Royal Infirmary, Leicester

Karen H Simpson FRCA, Consultant in Anaesthesia & Pain Management, St James's University Hospital, Leeds

J Robert Sneyd MD MA MB BChir FRCA, Reader in Anaesthesia, University of Plymouth Postgraduate Medical School, Plymouth

Andrew Vickers, Consultant Anaesthetist, Royal Lancaster Infirmary, Lancaster

Preface

Anaesthesia in developed countries is extremely safe. Death directly as a result of an anaesthetic mishap is rare and the cause is usually obvious. Post-operative nausea and vomiting (PONV), on the other hand, are very common after anaesthesia and surgery, and the cause is not clear but most likely is multi-factorial. Although rarely life-threatening, PONV is one of the commonest things that patients ask about pre-operatively and complain about post-operatively. Over the past ten years or so, since the advent of day surgery, PONV has become of increasing interest as study of morbidity after anaesthesia and surgery comes into focus. A key reason why patients cannot go home immediately after day surgery is PONV. Inpatients also are under pressure to go home as soon as practicable, and PONV may be a delaying factor.

As part of this increase in interest in morbidity has come, not before time, some would say, an increasing awareness that control of pain after surgery is an important factor. However, the indiscriminate use of opioids may contribute to PONV and more sophisticated approaches to post-operative pain relief are required. There are a plethora of drugs old and new, which have in pharmacological terms anti-emetic and anti-nausea properties. Are they effective in the 'real world of clinical practice'? In addition, claims are made for non-pharmacological interventions in PONV.

This book brings together experts in the field and will provide the reader with a comprehensive review of PONV. For simplicity, we have divided the presentations into three sections – *assessment*, *evidence and treatment,* and *multi-disciplinary approaches and strategies*.

In *assessment*, Drs Benton and Sneyd look at the epidemiology and risk of PONV. Paul Andrews brings the physiologist's view to bear on the mechanism of PONV and sets the stage for the rational use of drugs in relation to their sites of action. The multi-factorial nature of PONV leads one to the concept of a cascade of drugs and a plan for each patient depending on the circumstances. It is unlikely that any one strategy will prove effective for all patients and circumstances.

In *evidence and treatment*, Professor Harmer tackles the drugs and their side-effects, Dr Simpson provides an authoritative look at non-pharmacological intervention, and Professor Rowbotham reviews combination therapy and decisions for competing treatments. He also approaches the difficult scenario as what to do if current anti-emetic therapy fails. In this respect, if there is prolonged PONV after anaesthesia and surgery, a review of all therapies and drugs (including intravenous antibiotics) which a patient is taking should be undertaken to evaluate their role as potentially causative factors. Philip Howard reminds us of the considerable safeguards required in the preparation and administration of drugs seen from the standpoint of the pharmacist.

In *multi-disciplinary approaches and strategies*, Dr Vickers outlines the problems of PONV relative to inpatients and day-care patients. Fiona Dobson, an acute pain nurse specialist, Steve Haigh, a senior pharmacist, and Dr Greg Hobbs illustrate how the team approach may improve clinical outcome. Finally, Dr Hopkins points the way for further research. There are some exciting new classes of drugs on the horizon which may alter our perception of managing both PONV and pain together.

In the current age, where doctors and health professionals are increasingly overwhelmed by clinical information, we have aimed to provide a fully current, fully referenced text which is as succinct as possible but as comprehensive as necessary. Consultants and training grades in anaesthesia will find it of particular use as part of continuing medical education and specialist training, and we advance it explicitly as an excellent tool for these purposes. We anticipate, however, that the book will prove of not inconsiderable use to hospital nurses and pharmacists as a reference text, and to commissioners of health services as the basis for discussion and negotiation of health contracts with their practising colleagues.

In conclusion, we thank Glaxo Wellcome UK Ltd for the grant of educational sponsorship which helped organise a major national symposium on PONV at the Royal College of Anaesthetists, at which synopses of the constituent chapters of this book were presented.

Leo Strunin MD FRCA FRCPC
David J Rowbotham MD MRCP FRCA
Andrew Miles MSc MPhil PhD

PART 1

Assessment

Chapter 1

Epidemiological aspects of PONV and assessment of risk

Jennifer I Benton and J Robert Sneyd

Introduction

Post-operative nausea and vomiting (PONV) were first described in 1848 by John Snow (1848) within 18 months of the introduction of anaesthesia into Britain. The belief that anaesthetics alone were responsible for most cases of PONV persisted until 1916 when Flagg (1916) reported that post-operative vomiting may result from other causes, including pain, ovarian surgery, reflex responses and opioids. In 1956 Bellville *et al.* (1960) reported that choice of anaesthetic agent, the type of surgery and administration of anti-emetic were likely to influence the incidence and severity of PONV.

The incidence of PONV in adults is approximately 25 per cent, ranging from 5 to 75 per cent in published series (Burtles & Peckett 1957; Bonica *et al.* 1958; Bellville *et al.* 1960; Cohen *et al.* 1986, 1992). Review of the literature on individual factors contributing to PONV is complicated by lack of standardisation of the definitions of 'nausea' and 'vomiting' and frequently by the failure to control other factors which may contribute to PONV. The epidemiological factors of PONV can be divided into patient, surgical and anaesthetic factors. These are examined below.

Patient factors

Age and sex

In children the risk of PONV is commonly reported as almost twice that for adults (Vance *et al.* 1973; Cohen *et al.* 1990). However, few data exist to compare the incidence under controlled circumstances, i.e. with adults and children undergoing similar procedures with the same anaesthetic technique. There is an equal distribution of PONV between boys and girls until puberty (Vance *et al.* 1973; Rowley & Brown 1982). In adults women are 2–3 times more likely to suffer from PONV than men (Burtles & Beckett 1957; Bellville *et al.* 1960; Fahy & Marshall 1969; Muir *et al.* 1987; Zelcer & Wells 1987) until over 70 years of age where both sexes appear equally affected (Purkis 1964).

Previous PONV

In one study the incidence of PONV was three times greater in patients with previous PONV (Purkis 1964). Palazzo & Evans (1993) used logistic regression to develop a model predicting PONV in patients undergoing minor orthopaedic surgery. The factor receiving the greatest weight was a past history of PONV and the group at overall greatest risk were females with a history of PONV and motion sickness. The usefulness of attempting to predict PONV has recently been reviewed (Korttila 1998).

Motion sickness

Kamath *et al.* (1990) reported an increased incidence of PONV in those patients with motion sickness. Toner *et al.* (1996) confirmed a weak association. Our own investigation of gynaecological patients undergoing day-case diagnostic laparoscopy shows no relationship between motion sickness and PONV up to one week after surgery (unpublished data).

Phase of menstrual cycle

Reports of the menstrual cycle phase being linked to the risk of PONV are conflicting. Bellville (1961) reported that in adult females the highest incidence of PONV occurred during the third and fourth week of the menstrual cycle. Beattie *et al.* (1991) found it to be more common during the luteal phase (days 20–24), compared to the follicular phase (days 8–12) and the pre-menstrual phase (days 25–26), whereas Honkavaara *et al.* (1991) found the incidence to be greater during days 1–8. The incidence of PONV is lower in post-menopausal women (Purkis 1964).

Obesity

Although some authorities have suggested an excess of PONV in obese patients (Palazzo & Strunin 1984; Watcha & White 1992), this association is not generally accepted. Muir *et al.* (1987) studied 780 patients and found no relationship between body mass index and the incidence of PONV. Furthermore, the predictive equation of Palazzo & Evans does not include any independent term for body mass index or weight. To date, there is insufficient evidence to conclude that there is a relationship between obesity and PONV (Muir *et al.* 1987).

Surgical factors

Nature of operation

Since 1916 when Flaggs suggested an association between ovarian surgery and PONV, the wide discrepancies in reported incidences of PONV are usually reported in association with the surgery undertaken (Rowley & Brown 1982; Pataky *et al.* 1988).

Children

In children the procedure associated with the highest incidence of PONV is correction of squints, where it ranges between 40 and 88 per cent in children older than 2 years (Lerman *et al.* 1986; van den Berg *et al.* 1987; Warner *et al.* 1988; van den Berg *et al.* 1989; Lin *et al.* 1992) and tends to occur after mobilisation for up to 24 hours after surgery (Schreiner *et al.* 1992). No correlation has been demonstrated between the number of extra-ocular muscles repaired and the incidence of PONV (Smith & Manford 1974; Lerman *et al.* 1986).

Following adeno-tonsillectomy the incidence of PONV is 36–76 per cent (Rowley & Brown 1982; Puttick & van der Walt 1987; Yentis & Bissonnette 1991) and may be attributed to three mechanisms:

- blood in the upper gastrointestinal tract (Smith & Manford 1974)
- stimulation of trigeminal nerve afferents during surgery
- the administration of peri-operative opioids (Brown 1963).

Reflex stimulation through the auriculo-temporal branch of the facial nerve may lead to PONV after surgery to correct 'bat ears' (Vance *et al.* 1973). Hernia repair and orchidopexy have a reported PONV incidence of 54–58 per cent (Rowley & Brown 1982).

Adults

In adults abdominal, gynaecological and ENT surgery account for the highest incidence of PONV (see Table 1.1).

Table 1.1 Incidence of PONV after different surgical procedures in adults

Nature of surgery	*Incidence (%)*
Gynaecological laparoscopy (Madej & Simpson 1986; Hovorka *et al.* 1989)	40–77
Major gynaecological and hysterectomy (Pataky *et al.* 1988)	65–77
Therapeutic abortions and ovum retrieval (Pataky *et al.* 1988)	55
Dilatation and curettage (without vaginal packing or uterine evacuation) (Dundee *et al.* 1962)	25–36
Intra-abdominal, including intestine and gall bladder (Bonica *et al.* 1958)	70
Abdominal wall (Bonica *et al.* 1958)	15
Ear surgery (Vance *et al.* 1973)	47
Dental (Pataky *et al.* 1988)	16
Head and neck (Vance *et al.* 1973)	25–33

Length of operation

Several investigations have reported on the relationship between the duration of surgery and PONV but the results are conflicting and recent data scanty. Bellville *et al.* (1960) reported an almost 3-fold increase after longer procedures, whereas others found no correlation (Gold 1969).

Anaesthetic factors

Experience of anaesthetist

It has been 'known' for many years that the experienced anaesthetist has fewer patients who suffer from PONV than the inexperienced (Rubin & Metz-Rubin 1951; Bellville *et al.* 1960). This may be because inexperienced anaesthetists tend to maintain the patient at a deeper level of anaesthesia (Bellville 1961). In addition, manual inflation of the lungs by an inexperienced anaesthetist using a face mask prior to tracheal intubation has been associated with a higher incidence of PONV than when the procedure is carried out by an experienced anaesthetist (Hovorka *et al.* 1990). This may be due to inadvertent insufflation of the stomach with air. Other workers have also implicated mask ventilation as a cause of PONV (Dent *et al.* 1955).

Pre-medication

Centrally acting anticholinergics such as hyoscine and atropine may reduce the incidence of PONV (Mirakhur 1991), whereas glycopyrrolate, which does not cross the blood brain barrier, does not (Salmenpera *et al.* 1992). Recently, the use of benzodiazepine pre-medication has become common. The use of temazepam and diazepam in adults (Forrest *et al.* 1990; Kamath *et al.* 1990) and diazepam in children (Karlsson *et al.* 1990) has not been associated with PONV.

Anaesthetic agents

The induction agents methohexitone and etomidate are associated with a significant increase in PONV compared to sodium thiopentone and propofol (Clarke 1984).

Many studies have reported a reduced incidence of PONV when anaesthesia was induced or maintained with propofol; however, individual studies often lack statistical power. Meta-analysis is a statistical process whereby data from multiple studies are combined to yield an overall summary statistic (Chalmers & Altman 1995). For meta-analysis to be useful it is important for all relevant studies to be identified and for heterogeneity between studies to be investigated. Publication bias – the tendency for studies with positive results to achieve priority in publication over those with negative or neutral findings – is an important source of heterogeneity and has been blamed (Egger & Smith 1995) for the different conclusions reached by a meta-analysis of studies of intravenous magnesium after myocardial infarction and a subsequent mega-study, ISIS4. All data from meta-analysis must therefore be viewed with appropriate caution. Three groups have used meta-analysis to compare the incidence of nausea and vomiting after inhalational and intravenous maintenance of anaesthesia. Jobalia & Mathieu (1994) relied exclusively on a MEDLINE search and identified 28 studies covering 1,116 patients who were randomised to maintenance of anaesthesia with propofol or an inhalational agent. They reported that the odds ratios for PONV following maintenance with propofol were 0.29, 0.25 and 0.29 for vomiting, nausea, and 'nausea and vomiting' respectively. Tramer *et al.* (1997a) undertook a meta-analysis of 84 studies covering 6,069 patients randomised to intravenous induction or maintenance of anaesthesia with propofol, or 'other anaesthetics', which included inhalational anaesthesia as well as propanidid, midazolam or alphaxolone. They found that use of propofol as the induction agent was associated with a reduced risk of early nausea and vomiting (odds ratios of 0.45 and 0.47 respectively).When propofol was also used to maintain anaesthesia, the odds ratios were 0.34 and 0.25 for nausea and vomiting respectively within the first six hours after anaesthesia and 0.36 and 0.55 respectively beyond six hours. They also calculated the 'number needed to treat' (NNT) (Cook & Sackett 1995), i.e. the number of patients who would need to be given propofol anaesthesia to avoid one case of nausea or vomiting, as 4.7 and 4.9 respectively. A recent meta-analysis (Sneyd *et al.* 1998) reviewed 96 studies. Many of these studies had multiple treatment arms and after excluding the least-appropriate comparator groups, data from 5,214 patients were analysed. The odds ratios for nausea, vomiting, and nausea or vomiting were 0.38, 0.27 and 0.37 respectively, yielding an NNT of 8.1, 7.1 and 6.6 respectively. Sub-group analysis suggested that type of surgery, opioid usage, patient age and nitrous oxide usage did not affect the odds ratios obtained. When propofol was compared to sevoflurane and desflurane, the findings were similar to comparisons with older agents, i.e. the newer inhalational anaesthetic agents do not appear to reduce PONV (Sneyd *et al.* 1998).

Although no randomised mega-study has been undertaken definitively to address the benefits of intravenous anaesthesia, a large prospective study of 25,981 patients (McLeskey *et al.* 1993) in 1,772 hospitals revealed a low incidence (1.9 per cent) of PONV following propofol anaesthesia.

The association between induction and maintenance of anaesthesia with propofol and a reduced risk of PONV is now well established. However, the relative utility of this approach and other PONV reduction strategies has not been critically compared. Critics of intravenous anaesthesia point to the NNT and question whether this technique is a cost-effective method of reducing PONV (Tramer *et al.* 1997a & 1997b). Crucially, the interaction between different components of PONV remains uncertain, thus nitrous oxide alone is certainly emetogenic but this may not be the case when it is used as a component of a balanced anaesthetic (Hovorka *et al.* 1989; Sneyd *et al.* 1998).

Neuromuscular blocking and reversal agents

The neuromuscular blocking agents in current use have not been shown to have an effect on PONV. It was thought that the use of neostigmine to reverse muscle paralysis was strongly correlated with PONV (King *et al.* 1988); however, recent work suggests this is not the case (Hovorka *et al.* 1997; Nelskyla *et al.* 1998).

Peri-operative opioids

All agents that act at the μ-opioid receptor appear to cause nausea and vomiting, and attempts to separate this effect from analgesic efficacy have been unsuccessful. The role of opioids in PONV is unclear as intravenous techniques generally include an opioid but have a low incidence of PONV (Sneyd *et al.* 1998). These data suggest that the contribution of anaesthetic drugs to PONV is dominated by the choice of maintenance agent, with opioids acting as a less important factor.

Maintenance of anaesthesia with remifentanil subjects the patient to a period of intense μ-opioid receptor stimulation yet PONV is no more common than with other opioids which would normally be used at a much lower dose (after adjustment for potency). Perhaps the influence of opioids on PONV is determined by their presence in the conscious rather than the unconscious patient?

Anaesthetic techniques

Spinal anaesthesia

In a prospective study of 952 patients undergoing spinal anaesthesia the overall incidence of nausea was 18 per cent and vomiting 7 per cent (Carpenter *et al.* 1992). The addition of adrenaline to the local anaesthetic, blocks with a sensory level higher than the fifth thoracic dermatome, and hypotension were associated with the greatest risk of PONV. The use of ephedrine to minimise hypotension (Datta *et al.* 1982) and administration of 100 per cent oxygen (Ratra *et al.* 1972) have been reported to reduce intra-operative nausea and vomiting. Neither of these studies reported on PONV.

Regional techniques

When neural block of limbs with local anaesthetics was compared to spinal anaesthesia, the incidence of PONV was reduced for 24 hours (Dent *et al.* 1955; Bonica *et al.* 1958). This may reflect the different haemodynamic consequences of the two techniques.

Post-operative pain

Post-operative pain has been reported to increase the incidence of PONV after abdominal surgery (Andersen & Krohg 1976), and the administration of opioids to relieve the pain alleviated the nausea in 80 per cent of cases.

Post-operative fluids

The effects on PONV of timing of post-operative administration of oral fluids is unclear. Schreiner *et al.* (1992) have suggested a reduction of up to 50 per cent in PONV prior to discharge from hospital when oral fluids were withheld from children after adeno-tonsillectomy and strabismus surgery until they requested a drink but this strategy did not reduce the overall incidence of PONV over 24 hours, as many children vomited during the journey or at home. Van den Berg *et al.* (1987) reported that in adults and children who had undergone ophthalmic surgery, withholding oral fluids for at least four hours did not affect the incidence of PONV.

Conclusions

What should we do with this information? Patient and surgical factors are beyond the control of the anaesthetist, however, we can choose our anaesthetic technique. Risk of PONV is probably minimised by using propofol and an opioid or a regional technique, while avoiding nitrous oxide. Should we use intravenous anaesthesia for every case? Many clinicians are daunted by the apparent complexity and cost of intravenous anaesthesia and worry about peri-operative awareness. While these concerns may be ill founded, they must be respected. If prediction of PONV were a precise art, i.e. both sensitive and specific, then we could target our efforts at those patients at greatest risk. It is not enough to predict the risk in a population of patients because clinicians treat patients individually and, if predictions are to be useful, they must work at an individual level as well. When the Palazzo & Evans (1993) scoring system was tested prospectively in 400 patients, it was reasonably predictive of population risk, predicting an incidence of PONV of 36 per cent, when the actual incidence was 27.4 per cent (Toner *et al.* 1996). However, when the same model was used to define individual patients as predicted to have or not to have PONV, it was correct only 71 per cent of the time. Therefore, predictions for individuals are imperfect and those patients not identified as at risk may be denied techniques which could minimise their morbidity. Since we cannot predict risk for individuals, we can consider treating populations. The appropriateness of this strategy must balance the cost and risk of treating prophylactically that subset of the patient population who are in fact at low/no risk. At present we cannot reliably identify those individuals to whom treatment offers cost and risk but little or no benefit.

We are further hindered by the minimal data comparing different strategies. Does the addition of one or more prophylactic anti-emetics to an inhalational technique give a lower risk of PONV than an intravenous technique? Does the use of anti-emetics make an intravenous technique ‘even better’ or would they simply add risk of drug-related side-effects without reducing morbidity? At present we don’t know.

The patient, procedural and pharmacological factors associated with PONV have now been clearly defined and a framework for PONV studies established (Korttila

1992). Future work is needed to define the interaction of these factors and the cost-effectiveness of different strategies for reducing or preventing PONV.

References

Andersen R & Krohg K (1976). Pain as a major cause of post-operative nausea. *Can Anaesth Soc J* **23**(4), 366–9.

Beattie WS, Lindblad T, Buckley DN *et al.* (1991). The incidence of post-operative nausea and vomiting in women undergoing laparoscopy is influenced by the day of menstrual cycle. *Can J Anaesth* **38**(3), 298–302.

Bellville J (1961). Post-anesthetic nausea and vomiting. *Anesthesiology* **22**, 773–80.

Bellville JW, Bross IDJ & Howlans WS (1960). Post-operative nausea and vomiting. IV. Factors related to post-operative nausea and vomiting. *Anesthesiology* **6**, 186–93.

Bonica J, Crepps W, Monk M *et al.* (1958). Post-anaesthetic nausea, retching and vomiting. *Anesthesiology* **19**, 532–40.

Brown H (1963). The applied anatomy of vomiting. *Br J Anaesth* **35**, 136–45.

Burtles R & Peckett BW (1957). Post-operative vomiting: some factors affecting its incidence. *Br J Anaesth* **29**, 114–23.

Carpenter RL, Caplan RA, Brown DL *et al.* (1992). Incidence and risk factors for side effects of spinal anesthesia (see comments). *Anesthesiology* **76**(6), 906–16.

Chalmers I & Altman DG (ed.) (1995). *Systematic reviews.* BMJ Publishing Group, London.

Clarke RS (1984). Nausea and vomiting. *Br J Anaesth* **56**(1), 19–27.

Cohen MM, Duncan PG, Pope WD *et al.* (1986). A survey of 112,000 anaesthetics at one teaching hospital (1975–83). *Can Anaesth Soc J* **33**(1), 22–31.

Cohen MM, Cameron CB & Duncan PG (1990). Pediatric anesthesia morbidity and mortality in the perioperative period. *Anesthesia and Analgesia* **70**(2), 160–7.

Cohen MM, Duncan PG, Pope WD *et al.* (1992). The Canadian four-centre study of anaesthetic outcomes: II. Can outcomes be used to assess the quality of anaesthesia care? (see comments). *Can J Anaesth* **39**(5, Pt 1), 430–9.

Cook RJ & Sackett DL (1995). The number needed to treat: a clinically useful measure of treatment effect (published erratum appears in *BMJ* **310**(6986), 105) (see comments). *BMJ* **310**(6977), 452–4.

Datta S, Alper MH, Ostheimer GW *et al.* (1982). Method of ephedrine administration and nausea and hypotension during spinal anesthesia for cesarean section. *Anesthesiology* **56**(1), 68–70.

Dent S, Ramachandra V & Stephen CR (1955). Post-operative vomiting: incidence, analysis and therapeutic measures in 3,000 patients. *Anesthesiology* **16**, 564–72.

Dundee J, Micholl R & Moore J (1962). Studies of drugs given before anaesthesia. *Br J Anaesth* **34**, 527.

Egger M & Smith GD (1995). Misleading meta-analysis (editorial) (see comments). *BMJ* **310**(6982), 752–4.

Fahy A & Marshall M (1969). Post-anaesthetic morbidity in out-patients. *Br J Anaesth* **41**(5), 433–8.

Flagg PJ (1916). *The art of anaesthesia* 1st edn. Lippincott, Philadelphia.

Forrest JB, Beattie WS & Goldsmith CH (1990). Risk factors for nausea and vomiting after general anaesthesia. *Can J Anaesth* **37**(4), Pt 2, S90.

Gold MI (1969). Post-anaesthetic vomiting in the recovery room. *Br J Anaesth* **41**(2), 143–9.

Honkavaara P, Lehtinen AM, Hovorka J *et al.* (1991). Nausea and vomiting after gynaecological laparoscopy depends upon the phase of the menstrual cycle. *Can J Anaesth* **38**(7), 876–9.

Hovorka J, Korttila K & Erkola O (1989). Nitrous oxide does not increase nausea and vomiting following gynaecological laparoscopy. *Can J Anaesth* **36**(2), 145–8.

Hovorka J, Korttila K & Erkola O (1990). The experience of the person ventilating the lungs does influence post-operative nausea and vomiting. *Acta Anaesthesiologica Scand* **34**(3), 203–5.

Hovorka J, Korttila K, Nelskyla K *et al.* (1997). Reversal of neuromuscular blockade with neostigmine has no effect on the incidence or severity of post-operative nausea and vomiting. *Anesthesia and Analgesia* **85**(6), 1359–61.

Jobalia N & Mathieu A (1994). A meta-analysis of published studies confirms decreased post-operative nausea/vomiting with propofol. *Anesthesiology* **81**(3A), A33.

Kamath B, Curran J, Hawkey C *et al.* (1990). Anaesthesia, movement and emesis. *Br J Anaesth* **64**(6), 728–30.

Karlsson E, Larsson LE & Nilsson K (1990). Post-anaesthetic nausea in children. *Acta Anaesthesiologica Scand* **34**(7), 515–18.

King MJ, Milazkiewicz R, Carli F *et al.* (1988). Influence of neostigmine on post-operative vomiting. *Br J Anaesth* **61**(4), 403–6.

Korttila K (1992). The study of post-operative nausea and vomiting. *Br J Anaesth* **69**(Suppl.1), 20S–23S.

Korttila K (1998). Can we predict who will vomit after surgery? (editorial; comment). *Acta Anaesthesiologica Scand* **42**(5), 493–4.

Lerman J, Eustis S & Smith DR (1986). Effect of droperidol pretreatment on post-anesthetic vomiting in children undergoing strabismus surgery. *Anesthesiology* **65**(3), 322–5.

Lin DM, Furst SR & Rodarte A (1992). A double-blinded comparison of metoclopramide and droperidol for prevention of emesis following strabismus surgery. *Anesthesiology* **76**(3), 357–61.

McLeskey CH, Walawander CA, Nahrwold ML *et al.* (1993). Adverse events in a multicenter phase IV study of propofol: evaluation by anesthesiologists and post-anesthesia care unit nurses. *Anesthesia and Analgesia* **77**(4, Suppl.), S3–9.

Madej TH & Simpson KH (1986). Comparison of the use of domperidone, droperidol and metoclopramide in the prevention of nausea and vomiting following major gynaecological surgery. *Br J Anaesth* **58**(8), 884–7.

Mirakhur RK (1991). Anticholinergic drugs in anaesthesia. *Br J Hosp Med* **46**(6), 409–11.

Muir JJ, Warner MA, Offord KP *et al.* (1987). Role of nitrous oxide and other factors in post-operative nausea and vomiting: a randomized and blinded prospective study. *Anesthesiology* **66**(4), 513–18.

Nelskyla K, Yli-Hankala A, Soikkeli A *et al.* (1998). Neostigmine with glycopyrrolate does not increase the incidence or severity of post-operative nausea and vomiting in outpatients undergoing gynaecological laparoscopy. *Br J Anaesth* **81**, 757–60.

Palazzo MG & Strunin L (1984). Anaesthesia and emesis. I: etiology. *Can Anaesth Soc J* **31**(2), 178–87.

Palazzo M & Evans R (1993). Logistic regression analysis of fixed patient factors for post-operative sickness: a model for risk assessment. *Br J Anaesth* **70**(2), 135–40.

Pataky A, Kitz D, Andrews R *et al.* (1988). Nausea and vomiting following ambulatory surgery: are all procedures created equal? *Anesthesia and Analgesia* **67**, S163.

Purkis I (1964). Factors that influence post-operative vomiting. *Can J Anaesth* **11**, 335–53.

Puttick N & van der Walt JH (1987). The effect of premedication on the incidence of post-operative vomiting in children after ENT surgery. *Anaesthesia and Intensive Care* **15**(2), 158–62.

Ratra CK, Badola RP & Bhargava KP (1972). A study of factors concerned in emesis during spinal anaesthesia. *Br J Anaesth* **44**(11), 1208–11.

Rowley MP & Brown TC (1982). Post-operative vomiting in children. *Anaesthesia and Intensive Care* **10**(4), 309–13

Rubin A & Metz-Rubin H (1951). Effect of dramamine upon post-operative nausea and vomiting. *Surgery, Gynecol Obstet* **92**, 415–18.

Salmenpera M, Kuoppamaki R & Salmenpera A (1992). Do anticholinergic agents affect the occurrence of post-anaesthetic nausea? *Acta Anaesthesiologica Scand* **36**(5), 445–8.

Schreiner MS, Nicolson SC, Martin T *et al.* (1992). Should children drink before discharge from day surgery? *Anesthesiology* **76**(4), 528–33.

Smith BL & Manford ML (1974). Post-operative vomiting after paediatric adenotonsillectomy. A survey of incidence following differing pre- and post-operative drugs. *Br J Anaesth* **46**(5), 373–8.

Sneyd JR, Carr A, Byrom WD *et al.* (1998). A meta-analysis of nausea and vomiting following maintenance of anaesthesia with propofol or inhalational agents. *Eur J Anaesth* **15**(4), 433–45.

Snow J (1848). *On narcotism by the inhalation of vapours*. Royal Society of Medicine Services Ltd, London, 1991 (facsimile edition).

Toner CC, Broomhead CJ, Littlejohn IH *et al.* (1996). Prediction of post-operative nausea and vomiting using a logistic regression model. *Br J Anaesth* **76**(3), 347–51.

Tramer M, Moore A & McQuay H (1997a). Propofol anaesthesia and post-operative nausea and vomiting: quantitative systematic review of randomized controlled studies. *Br J Anaesth* **78**(3), 247–55.

Tramer M, Moore A & McQuay H (1997b). Meta-analytic comparison of prophylactic antiemetic efficacy for post-operative nausea and vomiting: propofol anaesthesia vs omitting nitrous oxide vs total IV anaesthesia with propofol. *Br J Anaesth* **78**(3), 256–9.

van den Berg AA, Lambourne A, Yazji NS *et al.* (1987). Vomiting after ophthalmic surgery. Effects of intra-operative antiemetics and post-operative oral fluid restriction. *Anaesthesia* **42**(3), 270–6.

van den Berg AA, Lambourne A & Clyburn PA (1989). The oculo-emetic reflex. A rationalisation of post-ophthalmic anaesthesia vomiting. *Anaesthesia* **44**(2), 110–17.

Vance JP, Neill RS & Norris W (1973). The incidence and aetiology of post-operative nausea and vomiting in a plastic surgical unit. *Br J Plastic Surgery* **26**(4), 336–9.

Warner LO, Rogers GL, Martino JD *et al.* (1988). Intravenous lidocaine reduces the incidence of vomiting in children after surgery to correct strabismus. *Anesthesiology* **68**(4), 618–21.

Watcha MF & White PF (1992). Post-operative nausea and vomiting. Its etiology, treatment, and prevention (see comments). *Anesthesiology* **77**(1), 162–84.

Yentis SM & Bissonnette B (1991). P6 acupuncture and post-operative vomiting after tonsillectomy in children (see comments). *Br J Anaesth* **67**(6), 779–80.

Zelcer J & Wells DG (1987). Anaesthetic-related recovery room complications. *Anaesthesia and Intensive Care* **15**(2), 168–74.

Chapter 2

Towards an understanding of the mechanism of PONV

Paul LR Andrews

Introduction

As anaesthesia and surgery have become progressively safer procedures, attention has focused on other consequences which may reduce quality of life and delay recovery (e.g. disturbed gut function (Herbert *et al.* 1999)), resulting in a longer hospital stay.

The treatment of PONV is still a major challenge for patient management, although advances have been and continue to be made in understanding its underlying mechanisms. This chapter will focus on some aspects of PONV to illustrate not only areas in which progress is being made but also areas of neglect and ignorance.

Why PONV?

The emetic system is remarkable in that it can respond to diverse chemical stimuli which are very unlikely to have been present in the environment during the course of evolution at least until recently. In the wild, nausea and vomiting subserved defensive functions to protect the body against toxins ingested accidentally with the food (Andrew 1993). A fundamental question to understanding PONV is to identify how particular elements of the operative environment can (unfortunately) trigger this defensive reflex.

The unpleasant sensation of nausea stops further ingestion of contaminated food (c.f. 'warning' function of pain) and, probably of greater importance, leads to the formation of a learned or conditioned aversion. This links the taste, smell or sight of the food to a memory of the sensation of nausea which it induced on the previous occasion. Such conditioned aversions may only require a single exposure for induction and can last for many years, if not a lifetime. Many of the readers of this chapter will be able to identify foods which made them ill, particularly as a child, and which they will still not eat.

Aversive responses may also be induced by stimuli in the clinical environment, with the best characterised example being the response to anticancer chemotherapy drugs, such as cisplatin. Patients who experience nausea and vomiting as a side-effect during the first or subsequent cycles of treatment may develop anticipatory nausea and vomiting with the prevalence being about 25 per cent (Morrow *et al.* 1998). This may take the form of the induction of nausea or even vomiting by the receipt of a hospital appointment card, the sight of the hospital, the smell of the hospital or even the sight of the staff involved in administration of the chemotherapy in a non-clinical setting (e.g. supermarket). While post-operative nausea is not usually as severe or protracted as anticancer chemotherapy-induced nausea and vomiting, it has the same potential for inducing aversive and anticipatory responses. Even if an aversion is not induced, it is likely that each time the emetic system is activated the organism 'learns' from the experience.

The function of vomiting is to forcibly expel material in bulk from the upper gastrointestinal tract. The vomiting response to ingested toxins is self-limiting, provided that it has been detected prior to absorption, in that the toxin responsible for initiating the response is removed by the act which it triggers (i.e. vomiting). In contrast, when the emetic stimulus is in the blood stream as is the case in many clinical situations (e.g. anticancer chemotherapy) vomiting will not remove it from the body and the response will be protracted with the duration depending upon metabolism and excretion (Andrews & Davis 1995).

To summarise, the reason why PONV occurs is that some feature(s) of the operative environment is able to activate one or more of the inputs to the emetic system, which itself evolved to eject toxins via the mouth and by the genesis of nausea and aversions to learn from the experience. The clinical importance of learning and plasticity in the emetic system (Andrews *et al.* 1990b) have been relatively neglected. Consideration should be given to taking a complete emetic history as each time the system is activated it will influence the subsequent response even if the stimulus is different.

Physiology of nausea and vomiting

Pathways for activation and integration of the emetic reflex

The majority of our knowledge of the pathways by which vomiting can be induced comes from studies of animal models (e.g. dog, cat, ferret, house musk shrew, but not rats, mice and rabbits, which do not vomit) and perhaps with the exception of the psychological and cerebral influences the same pathways operate in humans.

The pathways have been studied using retching and vomiting as endpoints, as nausea is difficult to study in animals (see below) but it can be induced by activation of the same pathways that can induce vomiting. However, while retching and vomiting are generated by brainstem mechanisms, the genesis of nausea requires the presence of higher brain regions.

Three major pathways by which the emetic reflex can be induced have been identified (see Andrews 1993 and Andrews & Davis 1995 for reviews):

- abdominal vagal afferents
- area postrema
- vestibular system.

Abdominal vagal afferents

The vast majority of axons in the abdominal vagi are afferent (approx. 80–90 per cent) conveying information from the gut to the brainstem (primarily the nucleus tractus solitarius) about the degree of distension and contractile activity of the muscle (mechanoreceptors) (Grundy & Scratcherd 1989) and features of the luminal environment, such as osmolarity, pH and the shearing of contents against the mucosa (chemoreceptors). These afferents play a role in the daily regulation of the gastrointestinal motor and secretory responses to food. Both types of afferent can induce emesis when appropriately triggered with the signal having intensity (high frequency) and temporal (prolonged activation) domains to prevent 'accidental' triggering of the emetic reflex. Using electrical stimulation which activates the axons synchronously, retching can be induced in the anaesthetised animal in less than 20 seconds (Andrews *et al.* 1990b).

A considerable body of experimental evidence shows that the activation of the vagal afferent signalling information from the mucosa is indirect via the release of neuroactive agents such as 5-hydroxytryptamine (5-HT) and cholecystokinin (CCK) from enteroendocrine cells (Grundy & Scratcherd 1989; Andrews & Davis 1995; Hillsey & Grundy 1998). It is proposed that systemic cytotoxic drugs (e.g. cisplatin) and radiation used in the treatment of cancer induce the exocytotic release of 5-HT from the enterochromaffin (EC) cells via the generation of free radicals and the influx of calcium ions. The 5-HT acts on 5-HT_3 receptors (a ligand-gated ion channel) located on vagal afferents terminating in close proximity to discharge the afferent and provide an emetic signal to the brainstem (Andrews & Davis 1995). The major site of action of the 5-HT_3 receptor antagonists (e.g. granisetron, ondansetron) used in the treatment of chemotherapy-induced emesis is on the peripheral vagal afferent terminals to block the effects of 5-HT (Andrews & Davis 1995). The role of other neuroactive agents in the induction of emesis by activation of vagal afferents has not been investigated but their involvement could account for the less than complete blockade of acute nausea and vomiting by 5-HT_3 receptor antagonists in some chemo- and radiotherapy patients.

Appropriate activation of the abdominal vagal afferents can readily induce retching and vomiting, while similar stimulation of the greater splanchnic nerve does not (Andrews *et al.* 1990b). The role of the splanchnic afferents in the genesis of nausea is unclear but these afferents convey noxious sensations and nausea is associated with pain (Desbiens *et al.* 1997). A recent study in humans has shown that sympathetic activation heightens the perception of experimental induced distension (Iovino *et al.* 1995). Sympathetic activation is associated with nausea and hence sympathetically mediated heightened perception could contribute to the epigastric awareness reported in nausea.

Experimental studies of the emetic reflex have provided evidence of plasticity (Andrews *et al.* 1990b). These observations come from experiments in which the acute section of the abdominal vagi but not the greater splanchnic nerves abolishes the emetic response to a particular challenge (e.g. radiation) indicating a critical role for the vagi. However, when animals are tested several weeks later with the same emetic stimulus, a response is present. There is some indication that the splanchnic afferents may mediate the response but in other studies section of the splanchnic nerves failed to abolish the response leading to the suggestion that it was mediated by the release of a substance from the gut, entering the circulation to act on the area postrema (see below) (Andrews *et al.* 1992; Makale & King 1993).

Area postrema

The area postrema is a circumventricular organ located at the caudal extremity of the floor of the fourth ventricle in the region of the obex (Leslie & Reynolds 1991). The blood brain barrier is permeable in this region making it structurally adapted for the detection of circulating substances, including peptides, from the gut. Ablation studies (including in humans) (Lindstrom & Brizzee 1962) have implicated the area postrema in emesis and have led to it being termed the 'chemoreceptor trigger zone' (CTZ) for emesis. This terminology has led to the erroneous assumption that any substance in the circulation which causes emesis must do so via the area postrema (Leslie & Reynolds 1992). The area postrema has been implicated by ablation studies in the emesis induced by opiate and dopamine receptor agonists but recent studies have suggested that the site of action is not the area postrema but receptors on dendrites of the subjacent nucleus tractus solitarius (NTS), which project into the area postrema. The area postrema may thus be envisaged as providing a window to the NTS and lesions of the area postrema would inevitably cause collateral damage to the NTS, the major site of projection of vagal afferents. The role of the area prostrema thus needs to be reassessed.

Vestibular system

The vestibular labyrinths provide the pathway for the induction of motion sickness (Koch 1993) with the disparity between the input from the visual and vestibular systems providing a potent signal. However, while blind people may become motion sick, those with severe bilateral labyrinthine damage do not. The function and evolutionary relevance (if any) of motion sickness is unclear but the vestibular input into the brainstem appears to be of importance in modifying the sensitivity of the emetic reflex. For example, head position in healthy volunteers has been shown to influence the emetic response to apomorphine acting via the brainstem (Isaacs 1957).

Other pathways

The emetic reflex can be activated from a number of other sites but they have been less well studied in contrast to the above inputs. Both nausea and vomiting can be induced by electrical stimulation of the discrete regions of the cerebral hemispheres (Sem-Jacobsen 1968). The natural stimulus for activation is not known but it appears likely that this is the route by which psychogenic stimuli induce nausea and vomiting. It is not known if any drugs act here to induce nausea and vomiting. A probable role for these cerebral outputs is to modulate the sensitivity of the brainstem mechanisms.

Nausea and vomiting can be induced by activation of a population of cardiac ventricular vagal afferents, auricular vagal afferents and pharyngeal afferents (Andrews & Davis 1995). They may also be induced by visual, olfactory and gustatory inputs but it is unclear whether this is a learned response.

Nausea

The subjective nature of the sensation of nausea has made it difficult to study the mechanisms involved in its genesis, particularly in animals. There are no objective measures of nausea in humans which do not rely on self-report by the patient. Production of the sensation obviously requires activation of neural pathways, which eventually project to areas of the cerebral hemispheres dealing with conscious sensations. The question remains as to how these pathways are activated and whether the visceral awareness (particularly abdominal) which accompanies nausea is direct or referred.

Studies using motion as the stimulus suggest that nausea is induced by lower levels of activation of the inputs to the emetic pathway(s) than are required to induce vomiting (Koch 1993). This model would be consistent with the 'warning' function of nausea. Attempts to understand the mechanisms underlying nausea and to identify objective markers have focused on the endocrine, gastric and autonomic nervous system-mediated changes which accompany it.

Endocrine changes

These can be divided into those which occur as a component of the response to a stressful stimulus and those which appear specific to nausea. In the latter category plasma vasopressin (ADH, AVP) is the best example (Nussey *et al.* 1988; Koch 1995, 1997). Massive (>50x maximal antidiuretic levels in some studies) increases in vasopressin, but not oxytocin, have been reported in close temporal association with the onset and continued presence of nausea induced by illusory self-motion, oral ipecac, systemic apomorphine, cholecystokinin and anticancer chemotherapy drugs (e.g. cisplatin). Unfortunately, there do not appear to be any studies in patients with PONV. Such studies would be of interest but care would be needed to control for the degree of hydration. One function of the ADH would be to promote fluid conservation in anticipation of the expected fluid loss which will occur if vomiting and diarrhoea ensue but the magnitude of the rise suggests that it may have other functions. The effects of high concentrations of ADH on the gut are not well described but, by analogy with its constrictor effect on vascular smooth muscle, some elevation in tone is likely. This could account for the diffuse abdominal sensations which accompany nausea if the motor changes activated abdominal visceral afferents. High levels of circulating vasopressin could also have an effect on the area postrema (see above) to activate pathways projecting from the nucleus tractus solitarius to more rostral parts of the brain, either generating the sensation of nausea or acting in concert with another input.

Gastric motor changes

The most consistent alteration in gastric physiology associated with the presence of nausea is an increase in the gastric electrical slow wave frequency from ~3cpm to 4–9cpm (Koch 1995; 1997). This has been extensively studied in subjects exposed to illusory self-motion (vection) where the frequency increased prior to the onset of reported nausea. Similar frequency increases have also been observed during the first trimester of pregnancy and in patients with diabetic or idiopathic gastroparesis, functional dyspepsia, peptic ulcer disease and those undergoing abdominal surgery. It is unclear whether the dysrhythmias contribute to the genesis of the sensation of nausea (via activation of afferents) or whether they are secondary to the complex endocrine (e.g. adrenaline, ß endorphin, ADH) or autonomic changes which accompany nausea and stressful events. One study of tachygastrias in patients following major abdominal surgery failed to show a difference between the patients with and without PONV (Clevers *et al.* 1992). This suggests that the tachygastrias are induced by features of the operative environment but do not cause PONV. The presence of tachygastrias may be a predisposing or priming factor for the induction of PONV, with additional factors required for its expression.

Autonomic nervous system-mediated changes

Many of the signs which accompany nausea are mediated by the autonomic nervous system (Andrews 1999a) and are indicative of a generalised autonomic arousal as might be expected due to the generally stressful nature of the experience. These include overt salivation frequently accompanied by repetitive swallowing (and aerophagy?), tachycardia, an increase in heart inter-beat interval variability, pupil dilatation, cutaneous vasoconstriction and sweating, giving rise to the pallor and the cold clammy feel of the skin. However, there is no evidence that any of the above give rise to the sensation of nausea, although they may contribute to the general discomfort of the patient.

In conclusion, the mechanisms underlying the genesis of nausea are relatively poorly understood, although recent imaging studies have demonstrated activation of the inferior frontal gyrus in subjects nauseated by vestibular stimulation or oral syrup of ipecac (Miller *et al.* 1996). Further imaging studies particularly in nauseated patients are required to identify if one particular region of the cerebral hemispheres is implicated.

Retching and vomiting

In contrast to nausea the mechanisms generating retching and vomiting and temporally related events are relatively well understood.

Shortly before the onset of retching preparatory changes have taken place in the gastrointestinal tract (Lang 1990; Lang *et al.* 1993). Relaxation of the proximal stomach occurs mediated by suppression of activity in vagal efferents supplying intrinsic cholinergic neurones and an increase in activity in the vagal efferents supplying the non-cholinergic, non-adrenergic intrinsic inhibitory neurones. The latter use vasoactive intestinal polypeptide and nitric oxide as their neurotransmitter. The relaxation is proposed to have three functions: to reduce emptying of potentially contaminated gastric contents into the duodenum; to place the proximal stomach in an optimum mechanical position for compression by the abdominal muscles and diaphragm during vomiting; and to accommodate refluxed intestinal contents.

Immediately prior to the initiation of retching a contraction is initiated in the mid-small intestine which sweeps retrogradely towards the stomach. This 'retrograde giant contraction' (RGC) is under vagal cholinergic control and can be blocked by atropine. The primary function of the RGC is to return intestinal contents, which may be contaminated, to the stomach from where they can be expelled by vomiting. It has also been proposed that pancreatic juice will enter the stomach by the RGC and may serve to buffer the acidic gastric contents prior to vomiting. The RGC probably accounts for the frequent presence of bile in the stomach. During surgery bile may also enter the stomach if gastroduodenal motility is disrupted. The irritant nature of bile may provide a further emetic drive by stimulation of the mucosal afferents.

Retching begins when the RGC reaches the stomach, marking the end of the prodromal or pre-ejection phase and the beginning of the ejection phase. However, the RGC is not essential for its initiation, as retching will occur even if the RGC is blocked either by atropine or abdominal vagotomy.

Retching is frequently referred to as 'unproductive vomiting' or 'attempts to vomit' and while both expressions are true, retching and vomiting are distinct but related processes (Koga & Fukuda 1990; Grelot & Miller 1996). During retching the anterior abdominal muscles (e.g. oblique, rectus and transverse abdominis muscles) and all parts of the diaphragm contract synchronously and rhythmically, whereas during vomiting there is more intense and prolonged activation of all the muscles except the perioesophageal (crural) diaphragm, which does not contract. In addition, during vomiting a retrograde contraction occurs in the striated muscle portion of the oesophagus and the upper oesophageal sphincter is widely opened by intense activation of the geniohyoid muscle (Minami *et al.* 1995; Grelot & Miller 1996). Thus the major expulsive force for vomiting is generated by compression of the stomach by contraction of the abdominal muscles and the descending diaphragm. During retching and vomiting a characteristic posture is usually adopted presumably to optimise the compression of the stomach and perhaps prevent strain of some muscle groups.

The function of retching is unclear and, as vomiting can occur without prior retching, it is clearly not an essential prerequisite. It has been proposed that retching helps overcome the antireflux barrier in the region of the lower oesophageal sphincter and to impart momentum to the gastric contents for expulsion. The factors regulating the number of retches preceding a vomit are unclear, although animal studies have shown that the number of retches is influenced by gastric volume, with low volumes increasing the number of retches preceding a vomit (Andrews *et al.* 1990a). What determines the transition from retching to a vomit is unclear, although blood gas levels have been implicated (Fukuda & Koga 1993).

The somatic and autonomic nervous system-mediated events are co-ordinated in the brainstem. The term 'vomiting centre' is a convenient shorthand term for the co-ordinating system but in reality the motor pattern is probably generated by a network of nuclei with perhaps the nucleus tractus solitarius and the central respiratory pattern generator playing predominant roles (Grelot & Miller 1996; Koga *et al.* 1998).

Emetic stimuli in the operative environment

The operative environment is complex, containing numerous potentially emetic stimuli. It is the interaction of these stimuli both with each other and with the individual patient which will determine whether a patient will experience PONV. Within this complex environment it is probable that some factors will have a greater effect than others and their removal would be expected to have a significant effect on the incidence of PONV. Epidemiological studies have identified a number of risk factors, such as volatile versus injected anaesthetics, the use of particular opiates and female gender (Palazzo & Strunin 1984; Andrews 1992).

In this chapter we will attempt to explain how some features of the operative environment may trigger this primitive protective reflex. It is not possible to review all the factors but they have been reviewed more extensively elsewhere (Palazzo & Strunin 1984; Andrews 1992; Watcha & White 1992).

Pre-operative factors

The previous emetic history of the patient will influence the response to subsequent emetic stimuli, as each time the emetic system is activated the patient will 'learn' from the experience. There is also a growing recognition that a patient's expectation of whether or not they will have emesis can influence the impact of anti-emetics (Eden & Zuk 1995). The use of such 'verbal-placebos' requires further investigation, particularly to identify the intrinsic mechanisms which are accessed by such interventions. Individual differences in emetic sensitivity, which suggest that there is likely to be a genotype which predisposes to an emetic phenotype, have probably been underestimated (Xu *et al.* 1993). There is some evidence for racial differences in emetic sensitivity and gender differences in emetic sensitivity are well described in humans, with females being more sensitive – although in some other species (e.g. the house musk shrew) the male is more sensitive to some emetic stimuli (Matsuki *et al.* 1997). In addition, 'environmental' factors, such as high alcohol intake, are protective against anticancer chemotherapy-induced emesis (D'Acquisto *et al.* 1986), but far less attention has been paid to the effects of smoking, which would be of particular interest as nicotine is a potent emetic. One factor which is overlooked and to which consideration should be given is the reason for the surgery, as it is likely that the emetic reflex is sensitised in patients who have symptoms of nausea and vomiting caused by their illness (e.g. gastrointestinal, central nervous system or labyrinthine disease) or condition (e.g. early pregnancy).

While all the above factors and others (e.g. glycaemic state, food, hydrational state) can predispose a patient to emesis during induction or post-operatively, they are not the cause of PONV, which must reside in stimuli to which the patient is exposed during surgery.

Peri- and intra-operative factors

The peri- and intra-operative environment provides a diverse range of mechanical and chemical emetic stimuli. Selected examples are discussed below.

Distension

Distension of the stomach and upper small intestine by a volatile anaesthetic could provide an emetic stimulus by activation of mechanoreceptors with afferents in the abdominal vagus. The most sensitive regions from which distension can induce nausea and eventually vomiting are those with little storage capacity such as the gastric antrum and the duodenum. During surgery gas is more likely to accumulate because of the marked reduction in motility which occurs. It is not known if the ability of the stomach to relax is impaired during anaesthesia and surgery. It is unlikely that distension provides a major stimulus, however, it may act as a facilitatory factor as, until the gas is voided, the nucleus tractus solitarius (see above) will be receiving a continuous input from the vagal afferents and distension, particularly of the gastric fundus, promotes relaxation of the lower oesophageal sphincter via a vago-vagal reflex.

Blood

In some forms of surgery (e.g. ENT) blood may enter the gastrointestinal tract and, although it has frequently been commented that blood is emetic, the mechanism has not been investigated directly. The effect of blood is more likely to be due to its chemical nature rather than distension. However, the emetic effect of blood is puzzling as in some cultures (e.g. Masai of Tanzania) ingestion of fresh blood taken directly from the jugular veins of cattle or sheep forms part of the diet (Tannahill 1996). If blood is emetic, the most likely source of the stimulus is the cellular components which contain, or have the ability to synthesise, a number of neuroactive agents (e.g. dopamine, 5-HT, ATP, prostaglandins, cytokines). Release of such agents in close proximity to the mucosa could activate nerve ending in the mucosa directly or indirectly by stimulating the release of mediators from the enteroendocrine cells in the mucosa (see above). As with distension, prolonged mucosal irritation by accumulated blood will sensitise the central pathways to other stimuli adding to the overall 'emetic burden'.

Opioids

Opioids have a wide spectrum of pharmacological effects depending upon the particular agent and the dose. Dose-response studies of morphine in animals have shown that at 'low' doses it is emetic, whereas at 'high' doses its emetic effects reduce (Thompson *et al.* 1992) and it can be shown to have anti-emetic effects blocking the response to other emetic agents (e.g. copper sulphate, apomorphine, cyclophosphamide) (Rudd & Naylor 1995). The type(s) of opioid receptor responsible for the different effects has not been identified but these appear to be due to an action on receptors in the area postrema/nucleus tractus solitarius in the brainstem. The anti-emetic effect of morphine and the emetic or pro-emetic effect of naloxone reported in several species, including humans, have been used as an indication that there is an 'anti-emetic centre' in the brainstem which can modulate the emetic reflex (Rudd & Naylor 1995). Identification of this region and its neurotransmitters would provide a novel target for anti-emetic drugs.

Clearly, morphine and related opioids could induce emesis by a direct central action if present when the patient emerges from general anaesthesia. However, opioids have other actions which could contribute to emesis by sensitising to other stimuli. For example, they can decrease gastric emptying, which may already be decreased by the use of muscarinic receptor antagonists, sensitise the vestibular system (opioids are more emetic in ambulatory patients), induce the release of ADH (see section on nausea, on page 17) and induce the release of 5-HT from the intestinal enterochromaffin cells (Racke & Schwoerer 1991). Each effect could induce nausea and vomiting if intense enough but, even if only activated to a low level, it would certainly contribute to the overall emetic burden to which the patient is exposed and perhaps sensitise to other emetic inputs.

It is perhaps timely to reassess the involvement of opioids in PONV as a number of agents other than morphine are in clinical use and understanding of opioid receptor pharmacology has improved as has clinical trials methodology. For example, a recent randomised, prospective and stratified study of patients undergoing strabismus or ENT surgery failed to demonstrate a statistically significant difference in PONV between patients who received low-dose opiates (fentanyl, sufentanil or alfentanil) or no opiate prior to induction of general anaesthesia (Kranke *et al.* 1998).

Anaesthetics

The recognition that neurotransmitter-gated ion channels (e.g. $GABA_A$, strychnine-sensitive glycine receptor, nicotinic acetylcholine receptor, ionotropic glutamate receptor) may be the molecular target for general anaesthetics suggests novel ways in which they may induce PONV (Peters & Lambert 1997).

A number of injectable (e.g. ketamine) as well as volatile anaesthetics (e.g. isoflurane, halothane) modulate the 5-HT_3 receptor, although not all general anaesthetics have the same action. A positive allosteric modulation could be a significant factor in the genesis of PONV (Parker *et al.* 1996). It is unlikely that such modulation of 5-HT_3 receptors alone accounts for PONV, as blockade by selective antagonists would be expected to be more efficacious than is the case. However, the relevant site for the modulation is probably 5-HT_3 receptors in the brainstem which are synaptically driven and, as the drugs used are competitive antagonists at the 5-HT_3 receptor, higher doses may be required than are used to block the emetic response to anticancer chemotherapy agents, where the major site is peripheral (see above). It would be of interest to investigate whether the emesis induced by some anaesthetics is more amenable to treatment with 5-HT_3 receptor antagonists than others.

Surgery

Surgery itself is perhaps the easiest stimulus to understand because it is evident that if the mechanical trauma of surgery activates one of the emetic pathways sufficiently, then emesis could result. However, this does not occur in normal clinical practice as the patient is anaesthetised and depending upon the type of surgery and national practice may have a neuromuscular blocking agent. These effects would be expected to be most marked during surgery but they probably persist into the post-operative period due to neuroactive agents released in response to local trauma (e.g. by damaged cells and axon reflexes). The unique nature of surgery in the experience of an animal should not be neglected as such trauma and manipulation of internal organs would only be experienced when an animal is being attacked!

Post-operative

It is in the post-operative period that nausea and vomiting occur. While the emetic stimuli are active during anaesthesia, the anaesthetic state suppresses but does not block the emetic pathway as intense activation of abdominal vagal afferents can induce retching even in deeply anaesthetised (i.e. absence of reflex withdrawal of a limb to a noxious stimulus) animals (Andrews & Davis 1995). From this it could be argued that the intra-operative emetic stimuli are not sufficiently intense. The suppression of the emetic reflex by general anaesthesia was used to reduce emesis in patients undergoing total body irradiation (Whitwam *et al.* 1978).

It is most likely that PONV results from an accumulation and persistence of the pre-, peri- and intra-operative factors but additional stimuli in the post-operative period may provide the final trigger. For example, on emergence from anaesthesia the patient will become aware of an altered state of consciousness and perception. While this may contribute to PONV, of arguably greater significance is motion.

During anaesthesia there is an absence of body, and particularly head, movement in comparison to sleep. Thus during surgery there will be an abnormally low input from the vestibular system which will become active as the patient is aroused, makes uncoordinated movements and is moved on a trolley, often in a semiconscious state.

Pharmacology of emesis and anti-emetics

Despite the large number of substances which are claimed to have anti-emetic properties, relatively little is known about the transmitters involved at key points in the emetic pathway. Care should be taken to distinguish between anti-emetics with direct effects blocking transmission at a critical point in the emetic pathway (e.g. NK_1 receptor antagonists, see below) and those which have an indirect action, such as alleviating gastric stasis (e.g. the 5-HT_4 receptor agonist effect of metoclopramide) (Andrews 1994).

Because an agent has an anti-emetic effect in one condition, it does not necessarily follow that it will have an effect in another condition; some consideration must be given to the underlying cause and the pathway activated. This can be illustrated by the 5-HT_3 receptor antagonists (Andrews 1994). These agents are very efficacious in the acute phase of anticancer chemotherapy-induced emesis because their primary site of action is to block the activation by 5-HT (released from the intestinal enterochromaffin cells by the chemotherapeutic agent) of the 5-HT_3 receptors located on the peripheral terminals of the vagal afferents. Any emetic stimulus acting via this pathway will have its effect reduced or blocked by a 5-HT_3 receptor antagonist. However, emetic stimuli acting via other mechanisms (e.g. motion, dopamine and opiate receptor agonists acting via the AP/NTS) will not be affected. 5-HT_3 receptors are present in the NTS but there is little evidence to implicate them in the anti-emetic effect of 5-HT_3 receptor antagonists at clinically relevant doses. The reduced efficacy of 5-HT_3 receptor antagonists in PONV, as compared to the acute phase of chemotherapy-induced emesis, suggests that activation of a pathway containing 5-HT_3 receptors plays a minor role in PONV. Based upon an understanding of the role of 5-HT and 5-HT_3 receptors in emesis (see above), it would be predicted that 5-HT_3 receptor antagonists would have the highest efficacy in abdominal and pelvic surgery when activation of the enterochromaffin cell–vagal afferent mechanism is expected to be greatest.

The transmitters most frequently implicated in the central emetic pathways are acetylcholine (acting on muscarinic M_3 receptors), histamine (acting on H_1 receptors) and dopamine (acting on D_2 and D_3 receptors). However, the site(s) at which they act are not known with any precision and they are relatively selective for particular types of emetic stimuli (e.g. H_1 for motion). However, blockade of one input (e.g. vestibular system, cortical arousal) may reduce the effect of activation of another input (e.g. vagal afferents) which is the primary site of action of the emetic challenge, thus providing some anti-emetic efficacy even if the anti-emetic is not targeting the primary input. This may account for the 'general' anti-emetic effects of agents, such as prochlorperazine, which have complex pharmacological actions (Rawlins *et al.* 1986).

It must be noted that many of the studies of anti-emetic efficacy were undertaken many years ago when trial design was often less rigorous than today. It would be of considerable interest to subject these studies to the type of analysis recently undertaken for the 5-HT_3 receptor antagonists to provide an accurate assessment of the involvement of each receptor type in PONV.

NK_1 receptor antagonists – the solution?

From the above discussion it is clear that identifying 'the mechanism' for PONV still lies in the future. One current approach to this and other forms of emesis where the precise mechanism is not known has been to identify 'broad-spectrum' or 'universal' anti-emetics. The ideal agent should be able to block nausea, retching and vomiting irrespective of the cause and without side-effects. In preclinical studies several receptor agonists have been shown to possess broad-spectrum anti-emetic effects. These include 5-HT_{1A} (Lucot 1995) and opioid (Rudd & Naylor 1995) receptor agonists. The approach which is being most actively pursued is blockade of the neurokinin-1 (NK_1) receptor, the preferred ligand for the peptide neurotransmitter substance P. Preclinical studies have shown that a number of selective NK_1 receptor antagonists have broad-spectrum anti-emetic effects when studied in a range of species (Watson *et al.* 1995b; Andrews 1999b). What is meant by this is that they can markedly reduce or block retching and vomiting induced by representative stimuli acting via the vestibular system, area postrema or abdominal vagal afferents (Table 2.1).

The site of action is proposed to be in the brainstem, most likely in the nucleus tractus solitarius – the convergence point for the emetic inputs; however, the link between the nucleus tractus solitarius and the 'emetic central pattern generator' has also been proposed (Watson *et al.* 1995a; Tattersall *et al.* 1996; Fukuda *et al.* 1998). While it is clear that the NK_1 receptor antagonists can block retching and vomiting, their effect on nausea cannot be assessed in animal studies. Early clinical studies of two NK_1 receptor antagonists (Hesketh *et al.* 1999; Navari *et al.* 1999) in anticancer therapy-induced emesis are encouraging and show that this class of agent may be particularly beneficial against nausea and vomiting in the delayed phase, which is particularly resistant to conventional anti-emetics and 5-HT_3 receptor antagonists. One preliminary study of an NK_1 antagonist against PONV in humans also showed encouraging results (Gesztesi *et al.* 1998). Further larger-scale, appropriately designed studies are required to assess whether the broad-spectrum anti-emetic activity shown in animal studies translates to the clinic. Whatever the outcome, important lessons have been learned from the study of this class of antagonist. For example, they have shown that it is possible to block emesis from three major pathways without producing any overt undesirable cardiorespiratory

Table 2.1 The preclinical spectrum of the anti-emetic effects on tachykinin NK_1 receptor antagonists

Stimulus	*Species*	*Compound*
Alcohol	*Suncus*	CP-99,994 (Chen *et al.* 1997)
Apomorphine	Ferret, dog	CP-99,994 (Watson *et al.* 1995a)
Cisplatin (acute/delayed)	Ferret, piglet, *Suncus*	CP-99,994 (Watson *et al.* 1995a; Rudd *et al.* 1996); GR205171 (Grelot *et al.* 1998); CP122,721 (Gonsalves *et al.* 1996); GR-203040 (Gardner *et al.* 1995); PD 154075 (Saito *et al.* 1998)
Copper Sulphate	Ferret, dog	GR203040 (Gardner *et al.* 1995); GR205171 (Grelot *et al.* 1998); CP-99,994 Watson *et al.* 1995a); CP-122,721 (Gonsalves *et al.* 1996); HSP-117 (Saito *et al.* 1998)
Cyclophosphamide	Ferret	GR-203040 (Gardner *et al.* 1995); GR205171 (Gardner *et al.* 1996)
Electrical vagal afferent Stimulation	Ferret/dog	CP-99,994 (Watson *et al.* 1995a); GR205171 (Fukuda *et al.* 1998)
Inhaled N_2O/isoflurane	*Suncus*	GR205171 (Gardner & Perren 1998)
Ipecacuanha	Ferret, dog	GR203040 (Gardner *et al.* 1995); GR205171 (Grelot *et al.* 1998); CP-99,994 (Watson *et al.* 1995a); CP-122,721 (Gonsalves *et al.* 1996)
Loperamide	Ferret	CP-99,994 (Watson *et al.* 1995a); CP-122,721 (Gonsalves *et al.* 1996)
Morphine	Ferret	GR203040 (Gardner *et al.* 1995); GR205171 (Gardner *et al.* 1996); HSP-117 (Saito *et al.* 1998)
Motion	*Suncus*, cat	GR203040 (Gardner *et al.* 1995); GR205171; CP-99,994 (Lucot *et al.* 1997)
Nicotine	*Suncus*	CP-99,994 (Tattersall *et al.* 1995)
Radiation	Ferret	GR203040 (Gardner *et al.* 1995); CP-99,994 (Otterson *et al.* 1997); GR205171 (Gardner *et al.* 1996)
Resiniferotoxin	*Suncus*	CP-99,994 (Andrews and Matsuki, unpubl. observ.)
Rolipram	Ferret	CP-99,994 (Andrews and Watson, unpubl. observ)

or behavioural effects. In addition, identification of the precise neuroanatomical site of action may point to a critical locus in the emetic pathway which is likely to have the same functionin humans even if substance P and NK_1 receptors are of less importance in this region in humans. If this is the case then it could contribute to efficacy differences which may be observed between humans (and perhaps other primates) and other animals.

References

Andrews PLR (1992). Physiology of nausea and vomiting. *Br J Anaesth* **69**, 2S–19S.

Andrews P (1993). Vomiting, a gastro-intestinal tract defensive reflex. *Pathophysiology of the gut and airways* **11**, 97–113.

Andrews PLR (1994). $5HT_3$ receptor antagonists and anti-emesis. In *$5HT_3$ receptor antagonists* (ed. FD King & GJ Sanger), pp.255–317. CRC Press, Boca Raton, USA.

Andrews PLR (1999a). Nausea, vomiting, and the autonomic nervous system. In *Autonomic failure* (ed. CJ Mathias & R Bannister), pp.126–35. Oxford University Press, Oxford.

Andrews PLR (1999b). Post-operative nausea and vomiting. In *Problems of the gastrointestinal tract in anaesthesia, the perioperative period, and intensive care* (ed. MK Herbert, P Holzer & N Roewer). Springer, Berlin-Heidelberg-New York (in press).

Andrews PLR & Davis CJ (1995). The physiology of emesis induced by anticancer therapy. In *Serotonin and the scientific basis of anti-emetic therapy* (ed. DJM Reynolds, PLR Andrews & CJ Davis), pp.25–49. Oxford Clin Comm, Oxford.

Andrews PLR, Bhandari P, Garland S, Bingham S, Davids CJ, Hawthorn J, Davidson HIM, Roylance R & Lane S (1990a). Does retching have a function? An experimental study in the ferret. *Pharmacodyn & Therap (Life Sci Adv)* **9**, 135–52.

Andrews PLR, Davis CJ, Maskell L *et al.* (1990b). The abdominal visceral innervation and the emetic reflex: pathways, pharmacology and plasticity. *Can J Physiol Pharmacol* **68**, 325–45.

Andrews PLR, Bhandari P & Davis CJ (1992). Plasticity and modulation of the emetic reflex. In *Mechanisms and control of emesis* (ed. AL Bianchi, L Grelot, AD Miller & GI King), pp.275–84. INSERM/John Libby Eurotext, Paris.

Chen Y, Saito H & Matsuki N (1997). Ethanol-induced emesis in the house musk shrew, *Suncus murinus*. *Life Sci* **60**, 253–61.

Clevers GJ, Smout AJPM, van der Schee EJ & Akkermans LMA (1992). Changes in gastric electrical activity in patients with severe post-operative nausea and vomiting. *J Gastrointest Mot* **4**, 61–9.

D'Acquisto RW, Tyson LB, Gralla RJ *et al.* (1986). The influence of a chronic high alcohol intake on chemotherapy-induced nausea and vomiting. *Proc Am Soc Clin Oncol* **5**, 257.

Desbiens NA, Mueller-Rizner N, Connors A-F & Wenger NS (1997). The relationship of nausea and dyspnea to pain in seriously ill patients. *Pain* **71**, 149–56.

Eden D & Zuk Y (1995). Seasickness as a self-fulfilling prophecy: raising self-efficacy to boost performance at sea. *J Appl Psychol* **80**, 628–35

Fukuda H & Koga T (1993). Hypercapnia and hypoxia which developed during retching participate in the transition from retching to expulsion in dogs. *Neurosci Res* **17**, 205–15.

Fukuda H, Koga T, Furukawa N, Nakamura E & Shiroshita Y (1998). The tachykinin NK_1 receptor antagonist GR205171 prevents vagal stimulation-induced retching but not neuronal transmission from emetic vagal afferents to solitary nucleus neurons in dogs. *Brain Res* **802**, 221–31.

Gardner C & Perren M (1998). Inhibition of anaesthetic-induced emesis by a NK_1 or 5-HT_3 receptor antagonist in the house musk shrew, *Suncus murinus*. *Neuropharmacology* **37**, 1643–4.

Gardner CJ, Twissell DJ, Dale TJ, Gale JD, Jordan CC, Kilpatrick GH, Bountra C & Ward P (1995). The broad-spectrum anti-emetic activity of the novel non-peptide tachykinin NK_1 receptor antagonist GR203040. *Br J Pharmacol* **116**, 3158–63.

Gardner CJ, Armour DR, Beattie DT, Gale JD, Hawcock AB, Kilpatrick GJ, Twissell DJ & Ward P (1996). GR205171: a novel antagonist with high affinity for the tachykinin NK_1 receptor, and potent broad-spectrum anti-emetic activity. *Regul Peptides* **65**, 45–53.

Gesztesi ZS, Song D & White PF (1998). Comparison of a new NK-1 antagonist (CP122,721). to ondansetron in the prevention of postoperative nausea and vomiting. *Anesth Analg* **86**, S32.

Gonsalves S, Watson & Ashton C (1996). Broad-spectrum antiemetic effects of CP-122,721, a tachykinin NK_1 receptor antagonist, in ferrets. *Eur J Pharmacol* **305**, 181–5.

Grelot L & Miller AD (1996). Neural control of respiratory muscle activation during vomiting. In *Neural control of respiratory muscles* (ed. AD Miller, AL Bianchi & BP Bishop), pp.239–48. CRC Press Inc, Boca Raton, USA.

Grelot L, Dapzol J, Esteve E, Frugiere A, Bianchi AL, Sheldrick RLG, Gardner CJ & Ward P (1998). Potent inhibition of both the acute and delayed emetic responses to cisplatin in piglets treated with GR205171, a novel highly selective tachykinin NK_1 receptor antagonist, in ferrets. *Eur J Pharmacol* **305**, 181–5.

Grundy D & Scratcherd T (1989). Sensory afferents from the gastrointestinal tract. In *Handbook of physiology*, Section 6: The gastrointestinal system; Vol 1. Motility and circulation; Part 1 (ed. JD Wood), pp. 593–620. Am Physiol Soc, Bethesda, USA.

Herbert MK, Holzer P & Roewer N (ed.) (1999). *Problems of the gastrointestinal tract in anaesthesia, the perioperative period, and intensive care*. Springer, Berlin-Heidelberg-New York.

Hesketh PJ, Gralla RJ, Webb RT, Ueno W, DelPrete S, Bachinsky ME, Dirlam NL, Stack CB & Silberman SL (1999). Randomized Phase II study of the neurokinin 1 receptor antagonist CJ-11,974 in the control of cisplatin-induced emesis. *J Clin Onc* **17**, 338–43.

Hillsley K & Grundy D (1998). Sensitivity to 5-hydroxytryptamine in different afferent subpopulations within mesenteric nerves supplying the rat jejunum. *J Physiol* **509**(3), 717–27.

Iovino P, Azpiroz F, Domingo E & Malagelada J-R (1995). The sympathetic nervous system modulates perception and reflex responses to gut distention in humans. *Gastroenterology* **108**, 680–6.

Isaacs B (1957). The influence of head and body position on the emetic action of apomorphine in man. *Clinical Science* **16**, 215–21.

Koch KL (1993). Motion sickness. In *The handbook of nausea and vomiting* (ed. M Sleisenger), pp.43–60. Parthenon Publishing Group, New York, USA.

Koch KL (1995). Approach to the patient with nausea and vomiting. In *Textbook of gastroenterology* 2nd edn (ed. T Yamada), pp.731–49. JB Lippincott Co, Philadelphia, USA.

Koch KL (1997). A noxious trio – nausea, gastric dysrhythmias and vasopressin. *Neurogastroenterology and Motility* **9**, 141–2.

Koga T & Fukuda H (1990). Characteristic behavior of the respiratory muscles, esophagus, and external anal and urethral sphincters during straining, retching, and vomiting in the decerebrate dog. *Jpn J Physiol* **40**, 789–807.

Koga T, Qu R & Fukuda H (1998). The central pattern generator for vomiting may exist in the reticular area dorsomedial to the retrofacial nucleus in dogs. *Exp Brain Res* **118**, 139–47.

Kranke P, Apfel CC, Papenfuss T, Meyer F, Sefrin P & Roewer N (1998). Influence of low-dose opioids for induction of inhalational anaesthesia on postoperative nausea and vomiting. *AINS* **9**, 531–634.

Lang IM (1990). Digestive tract motor correlates of vomiting and nausea. *Can J Physiol Pharmacol* **68**, 242–53.

Lang IM, Sarna SK & Dodds WJ (1993). Pharyngeal, esophageal, and proximal gastric responses associated with vomiting. *Am J Physiol* **265**, G963–72.

Leslie RA & Reynolds DJM (1991). The area postrema and vomiting, how important is serotonin? In *Current aspects of the neurosciences* (ed. NN Osborne) pp. 79–101. Macmillan, Basingstoke.

Leslie RA & Reynolds DJM (1992). Functional anatomy of the emetic circuitry in the brainstem. In *Mechanisms and control of emesis* (ed. AL Bianchi, L Grelot, AD Miller & GL King), pp.19–27. Colloque INSERM/John Libbey Eurotext Ltd, Paris, Montrouge, France.

Lindstrom PA & Brizzee KR (1962). Relief of intractable vomiting from surgical lesions in the area postrema. *J Neurosurg* **19**, 228–36.

Lucot JB (1995). 5-HT_{1A} receptor agonists as anti-emetics. In *Serotonin and the scientific basis of anti-emetic therapy* (ed. DJM Reynolds, PLR Andrews & CJ Davis) pp.222–7. Oxford Clin Comm, Oxford.

Lucot JB, Obach RS, McLean S & Watson JW (1997). The effect of CP-99,994 on the responses to provocative motion in the cat. *Br J Pharmacol* **120**, 116–20.

Makale MT & King GL (1993). Plasticity of autonomic control of emesis in irradiated ferrets. *Am J Physiol* **265**, R1092–9.

Matsuki N, Wang C-H, Okada F, Tamura M, Ikegaya Y, Lin S-C, Hsu Y-N, Chaung L-J, Chen S-J & Saito H (1997). Male/female differences in drug-induced emesis and motion sickness in *Suncus murinus*. *Pharmacol Biochem Behavior* **57**, 721–5.

Miller AD, Rowley HA, Roberts TPL & Kucharczyk J (1996). Human cortical activity during vestibular- and drug-induced nausea detected using MSI. *Ann N Y Acad Sci* **781**, 670–2.

Minami M, Endo T, Nemoto M, Hamaue N, Hirafuji M, Monama Y, Yajima T, Yoshioka M & Saito H (1995). The physiology of emesis induced by anticancer therapy. In *Serotonin and the scientific basis of anti-emetic therapy* (ed. DJM Reynolds, PLR Andrews & CJ Davis) pp.68–83. Oxford Clin Comm, Oxford.

Morrow GR, Roscoe JA, Kirshner JJ, Hynes HE & Rosenbluth RJ (1998). Anticipatory nausea and vomiting in the era of 5-HT_3 antiemetics. *Supportive Care in Cancer* **6**, 244–7.

Navari RM, Reinhardt RR, Gralla RJ, Kris MG, Hesketh PJ, Khojasteh A, Kindler H, Grote TH, Pendergrass K, Grunberg SM, Carides AD & Gertz BJ (1999). Reduction of cisplatin-induced emesis by a selective neurokinin-1 receptor antagonist. *New England J Med* **340**, 190–5.

Nussey SS, Hawthorn J, Page SR, Ang VTY & Jenkins JS (1988). Responses of plasma oxytocin and arginine vasopressin to nausea induced by apomorphine and ipecacuanha. *Clin Endocrinol* **28**, 297–304.

Otterson MF, Leming SC & Moulder JE (1997). Central NK1 receptors mediate radiation induced emesis. *Gastroenterology* **112**, A801.

Palazzo MGA & Strunin L (1984). Anaesthesia and emesis. I: Etiology. *Can Anaesth Soc J* **31**, 178–87.

Parker RMC, Bentley KR & Barnes NM (1996). Allosteric modulation of 5-HT_3 receptors: focus on alcohols and anaesthetic agents. *TIPS* **17**, 95–9.

Peters JA & Lambert JJ (1997). Anesthetics in a bind? *TIPS* **18**, 454–5.

Racke K & Schwoerer H (1991). Regulation of serotonin release from the intestinal mucosa. *Pharmacology Research* **23**, 13–25.

Rawlins MD, Taylor WB & Bateman DN (1986). Rational approaches to therapy for nausea and vomiting: two common solutions. In *Nausea and vomiting: mechanisms and treatment* (ed. CJ Davis, Lake-Bakaar & DG Grahame-Smith), pp.167–171. Springer-Verlag, Berlin.

Rudd JA & Naylor RJ (1995). Opioid receptor involvement in emesis and anti-emesis. In *Serotonin and the scientific basis of anti-emetic therapy* (ed. DJM Reynolds, PLR Andrews & CJ Davis) pp. 208–21. Oxford Clin Comm, Oxford.

Rudd JA, Jordan CC & Naylor RJ (1996). The action of the NK_1 tachykinin receptor antagonist, CP 99,994 in antagonizing the acute and delayed emesis induced by cisplatin in the ferret. *Br J Pharmacol* **119**, 931–6.

Saito R, Suehiro Y, Ariumi H, Migita K, Hori N, Hashiguchi T, Sakai M, Saeki M, Takano Y & Kamiya H-O (1998). Anti-emetic effects of a novel NK-1 receptor antagonist HSP-117 in ferrets. *Neurosci Let* **254**, 169–72.

Sem-Jacobsen CW (1968). *Depth electrographic stimulation of the human brain and behavior.* Thomas, Springfield (Ill), USA.

Singh L, Field MJ, Hughes J, Kuo B-S, Suman-Chauhan N, Tuladhar BR, Wright DS & Naylor RJ (1997). The tachykinin NK_1 receptor antagonist PD 154075 blocks cisplatin-induced delayed emesis in the ferret. *Eur J Pharmacol* **321**, 209–16.

Tannahill R (1996). *Flesh and blood. A history of the cannibal complex.* Abacus, London.

Tattersall FD, Rycroft W, Marmont N, Cascieri M, Hill RG & Hargreaves RJ (1995). Enantiospecific inhibition of emesis induced by nicotine in the house musk shrew (*Suncus murinus*) by the $Neurokinin_1$ (NK_1) receptor antagonist CP-99,994. *Neuropharmacology* **34**, 1697–9.

Tattersall FD, Rycroft W, Francis B, Pearce D, Merchant K, MacLeod AM, Ladduwahetty T, Keown L, Swain C, Baker R, Cascieri M, Ber E, Metzger J, MacIntyre DE, Hill RG & Hargreaves RJ (1996). Tachykinin NK_1 receptor antagonists act centrally to inhibit emesis induced by the chemotherapeutic agent cisplatin in ferrets. *Neuropharmacology* **35**, 1121–9.

Thompson PI, Bingham S, Andrews PLR, Patel N, Joel SP & Slevin ML (1992). Morphine 6-glucuronide: a metabolite of morphine with greater emetic potency than morphine in the ferret. *Br J Pharmacol* **106**, 3–8.

Watcha MF & White PF (1992). Postoperative nausea and vomiting – its etiology, treatment and prevention. *Anesthesiology* **77**, 162–84.

Watson JW, Gonsalves SF, Fossa AA, McLean S, Seeger T, Obach S & Andrews PLR (1995a). The anti-emetic effects of CP-99,994 in the ferret and the dog: role of the NK_1 receptor. *Br J Pharmacol* **115**, 84–94.

Watson JW, Nagahisa A, Lucot JB & Andrews PLR (1995b). The tachykinins and emesis: towards complete control? In *Serotonin and the scientific basis of anti-emetic therapy* (ed. DJM Reynolds, PLR Andrews & CJ Davis) pp. 233–8. Oxford Clin Comm, Oxford.

Whitwam JG, Morgan M, Owen JR, Goolden AWG, Spiers ASD, Goldman JM & Gordon-Smith EC (1978). General anaesthesia for high-dose total body irradiation. *Lancet* **1**, 128–9.

Xu LH, Koch KL, Summy-Long J, Stern RM, Seaton JF, Harrison TS, Demers LM & Bingaman S (1993). Hypothalamic and gastric myoelectrical responses during vection-induced nausea in healthy Chinese subjects. *Am J Physiol* **265**, E578–84.

PART 2

Evidence and treatment

Chapter 3

Pharmacological intervention in PONV: medical evidence for anti-emetic therapy and review of side-effect profiles

Michael Harmer

Introduction

The basis for the pharmacological control of PONV centres around the perceived mechanisms and receptors involved in the sensory, processing and motor actions responsible for its production. The proposed mechanisms involved in this process are ever-evolving, as we gain a better understanding of the interrelationships between physical, chemical and emotional sensory inputs that result in the processes of vomiting and nausea. It has equally become apparent that the mechanisms cannot be the same for the two modalities and that they are not of necessity linked – with nausea possible without vomiting or retching (an unproductive vomiting act) and vice versa.

Sensory inputs

As regards the specific area of PONV, it is probably acceptable to use a simple scheme of receptor interaction to explain why certain drugs may lead to PONV while others may reduce or eliminate it. The main afferent inputs that may stimulate PONV are shown in Figure 3.1. Although the vomiting centre has little anatomical meaning, it is a physiological concept that has been accepted as a representation of the central processing unit for vomiting (though possibly not for nausea). Further details of the physiology of PONV can be found in Chapter 2.

The main afferent inputs are: opioids, anaesthetic agents, vestibular and oropharyngeal stimulation, gastrointestinal receptors, and psychological inputs. Many of these inputs are influenced by anaesthesia or the peri-operative period.

Opioids and pain

Opioids are potent stimulators of nausea and vomiting and a common component of most general anaesthetics. They are also widely used in the post-operative period to treat pain. Avoidance may be helpful but an alternative analgesic regimen must be employed as pain itself is a potent stimulator of nausea and vomiting. The move in recent years towards an increased use of regional techniques for post-operative pain management has led to some improvements.

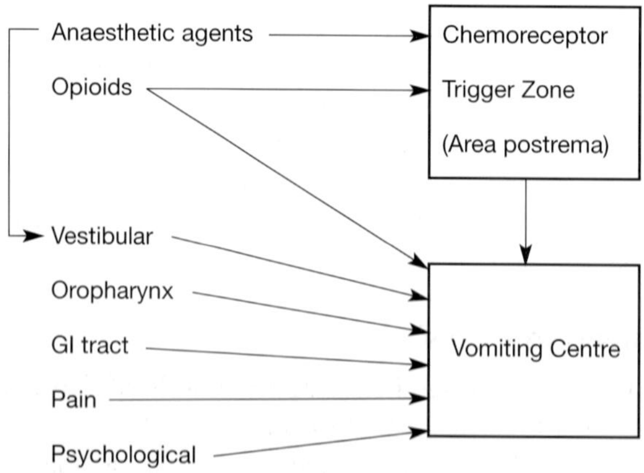

Figure 3.1 Afferent inputs involved in PONV

Anaesthetic agents

Many of the older agents such as ether and methohexitone were well recognised as potent stimulators of PONV. However, even currently used agents such as etomidate are known to cause PONV and, unless specifically indicated on other grounds, might sensibly be avoided in routine practice. In addition, nitrous oxide has been incriminated to some extent, with the mechanism probably relating to increases in air spaces subsequent upon it replacing nitrogen; thus there may be gut distension or increased middle-ear pressure. Finally, the use of neostigmine to reverse the effects of neuromuscular block has been linked to PONV. Modern neuromuscular blocking agents are often used in infusions and allowed to 'wear off' rather than needing reversal.

Vestibular and oropharyngeal stimulation

In addition to any effect of nitrous oxide on the middle ear, anaesthesia almost certainly sensitises the vestibular apparatus. The handling of patients in the immediate post-operative period with sudden changes of position and direction of movement is very likely to cause vestibular stimulation and subsequent PONV. Equally, the persistent use of pharyngeal suctioning, often with a rigid sucker, can have a profound stimulating effect on the vomiting process.

Gastrointestinal inputs

Although it may seem self-evident that a patient with a full stomach is more likely to suffer PONV than a starved patient, it may not be quite that simple, as there is some evidence that small quantities of clear fluid, rather than being detrimental, may be advantageous in promoting gastric emptying and hence in reducing the incidence (or volume) of vomiting.

Psychological inputs

The peri-operative patient undergoes a wide range of psychological experiences, including fear, anxiety, depression, elation, relief and pain. Allaying of any, or all, of these may help considerably in reducing the incidence of PONV. In the patient where clear explanation and discussion does not work, there may be a place for an anxiolytic. Thus careful, thoughtful peri-operative care can do much to reduce the necessity for prevention or treatment strategies.

Receptors involved in PONV

The pharmacology that has evolved for the management of PONV has centred largely upon the receptors thought to be involved. Much of the evidence upon which these receptors have been identified has come from animal models or from extrapolation from other areas of clinical practice in which nausea and vomiting are common problems. This may lead to some inconsistencies as there is not a good animal model for vomiting and the afferent inputs involved in such areas as chemotherapy may be very different to those in PONV. However, it is generally accepted that a number of receptors are involved in nausea and vomiting (Table 3.1).

Drugs used in the prevention and treatment of PONV

Drug therapy is based upon the receptor types believed to be involved in PONV and so is basically divided into: antidopaminergic, anticholinergic, antihistaminic and antiserotonergic drugs. These are reviewed below.

Antidopaminergic drugs

These drugs exhibit a range of activity at the dopaminergic receptor as well as having other effects. For example, metoclopramide has prokinetic effects, droperidol has sedative and autonomic effects, while prochlorperazine has hypnotic properties. As a group, they have been used for PONV for many years.

Table 3.1 Receptors involved in the process of PONV

Receptor type	*Site of action*
Dopamine Opioid 5-HT_3	Chemoreceptor trigger zone (Area postrema)
Cholinergic Histamine Opioid NK_1	Vomiting centre

Metoclopramide

Metoclopramide is a substituted benzamide first developed in the early 1960s. Its main action as an antidopaminergic is on the chemoreceptor trigger zone and it has prokinetic effects in enhancing gastric and upper intestinal motility. Metoclopramide also has some weak serotonin receptor activity (in particular 5-HT_3).

In his review of current management of PONV, Rowbotham (1992) identified a wide range of efficacy for metoclopramide, with a number of studies where metoclopramide was not considered statistically to be any better than placebo.

Scrutiny of the more recent randomised, controlled studies of metoclopramide in PONV have shown a very similar picture (Table 3.2). The wide variability in patient type, operation type, definition of PONV and design of studies makes comparison between different studies meaningless.

The incidence of vomiting ranges from 24 to 71 per cent in a variety of studies involving different types of surgery, patients and hospital setting (inpatient versus outpatient). As such, it is difficult to differentiate one aspect from another. However, it is interesting to note that two of the studies shown in Table 3.2 were placebo-controlled studies where metoclopramide showed no significant difference to placebo. Thus, one is left with a very similar impression to that of Rowbotham (1992) that metoclopramide in adults has a limited role as an anti-emetic in the peri-operative period, though it may have a place on account of its prokinetic effects.

There have been very few studies in children with the only placebo-controlled study (Scuderi *et al.* 1997) showing an incidence of vomiting of 32 per cent which was not statistically different from placebo.

Side-effects. The most important side-effects of metoclopramide are extrapyramidal reactions. These are more common in young female patients with a proposed incidence of 1 in 5,000 in the 12–19 years age range (Bateman *et al.* 1965). Sedation occurs in approximately 10 per cent of patients receiving long-term therapy (Harrington *et al.* 1983) but is seldom a problem when used for the treatment of PONV. Some authors have reported restlessness, agitation and akathisia after normal doses of metoclopramide (Dundee & Clarke 1973; Caldwell *et al.* 1987). Metoclopramide has also been associated with significant decreases of blood pressure (Pegg 1980) and increases in heart rate (Ellis & Spence 1970). It is thus recommended that intravenous metoclopramide should be given over 1–2 minutes.

The overall impression of metoclopramide in clinical practice is shown in Table 3.3.

Alizapide

Alizapide has only been studied once but was found to be effective (Stienstra *et al.* 1997) being comparable to droperidol and ondansetron (see below).

Table 3.2 Summary of recent studies on metoclopramide

Reference	*Type of patient*	*Type of surgery*	*Type of study (comparators)*	*Incidence of PONV (%)*
Lacroix *et al.* (1996)	Adults	General surgery	Prevention R, DB (droperidol, propofol)	24
Watts (1996)	Adults	Day case laparoscopic	Prevention R (ondansetron, cyclizine)	24
Fujii *et al.* (1998c)	Adult females	Breast surgery	Prevention R, DB, PC* (droperidol, granisetron)	43
Fujii *et al.* (1998d)	Adults	Middle ear surgery	Prevention R, DB (droperidol, granisetron)	53
Fujii *et al.* (1997)	Adult females with motion sickness	Major gynaecology	Prevention R, DB, PC* (droperidol, ondansetron)	57
Diemunsch *et al.* 1997	Adults	General	Treatment R, DB (ondansetron)	59
Fujii *et al.* (1998a)	Adult females with previous PONV	Major gynaecology	Prevention R, DB (droperidol, granisetron)	60
Nagiub *et al.* (1996)	Adults	Laparoscopic cholecystectomy	Prevention R, DB, PC* (droperidol, tropisetron, granisetron)	71
Scuderi *et al.* (1997)	Child	Outpatient strabismus	Prevention R, DB, PC* (droperidol, ondansetron)	32

R = randomised; DB = double blind; PC = placebo controlled; * = no difference to placebo; ** = significant difference to placebo

Table 3.3 Overall impression of metoclopramide

Benefits	*Drawbacks*
Widely used in clinical practice	Limited efficacy (?any better than placebo)
Useful prokinetic effects	Extrapyramidal side-effects
	Possible problems with gastrointestinal surgery

Droperidol

Droperidol is a butyrophenone and within the same family as major psychotrophic drugs such as haloperidol. Droperidol is a known potent neuroleptic and was developed for use in such a role. However, used in small doses, less than 5 mg (and often as little as 0.25 mg), it has been shown to have anti-emetic properties. A review of recent randomised, controlled studies in which droperidol has been used is presented in Table 3.4.

The incidence of vomiting in these adult studies shows a huge range from 4 to 57 per cent for a wide variety of operations and other variables. Three studies were placebo-controlled and in two, droperidol was statistically better than the placebo.

There have been two recent placebo-controlled studies in children (Scuderi *et al.* 1997; Goodarzi 1998), with a huge difference in the incidence of vomiting. Both studies showed droperidol to be better than placebo and in Scuderi's study, droperidol was deemed comparable to ondansetron in the immediately post-operative period, although subsequent measurements could not detect any difference.

In addition to its use as a prophylactic agent, droperidol has been used as an adjunct to patient-controlled analgesia. Using such a technique, Walder and Aitkenhead (1995) found an overall PONV incidence of 40 per cent in patients who had undergone major gynaecological surgery. However, the actual dose that is effective is open to debate as Lamond *et al.* (1998) could find no difference in effect for a bolus dose range of 0.05–0.2 mg.

Side-effects. The most common side-effect is delay in recovery caused by sedation. This is more likely with larger doses but can occasionally occur even with lower doses. Extrapyramidal reactions are also a recognised problem. Anxiety (Thorpe & Smith 1996) and akathisia (Foster *et al.* 1996) have been reported after relatively small doses of droperidol. These problems seem to occur some time after surgery and have led to concerns over the use of droperidol for day-case surgery.

The overall impression of droperidol in clinical practice is shown in Table 3.5.

Haloperidol

Haloperidol, although predominantly used as a major psychotrophic tranquilliser, has anti-emetic qualities (Judkins & Harmer 1982) when given orally as a pre-medicant.

Table 3.4 Summary of recent studies on droperidol

Reference	*Type of patient*	*Type of surgery*	*Type of study (comparators)*	*Incidence of PONV (%)*
Lacroix (1996)	Adults	General surgery	Treatment R, DB (propofol, metoclopramide)	4
Maestre *et al.* (1997)	Adults	Ambulatory	Prevention R, DB, PC* (metoclopramide, ondansetron)	6
Gan *et al.* (1994)	Adults	Hip and knee replacement	Prevention R, DB, PC** (ondansetron)	18
Loo *et al.* (1997)	Adult females	Minor gynaecology	Prevention R (droperidol + metoclopramide)	23
Fujii *et al.* (1998c)	Adult females	Breast surgery	Prevention R, DB, PC* (metoclopramide, granisetron)	37
Fujii *et al.* (1998d)	Adults	Middle ear surgery	Prevention R, DB (metoclopramide, granisetron)	46
Fujii *et al.* (1997)	Adult females with history of motion sickness	Major gynaecology	Prevention R, DB, PC** (metoclopramide, granisetron)	50
Fujii *et al.* (1998a)	Adult females with history of PONV	Major gynaecology	Prevention R, DB (metoclopramide, granisetron)	57
Scuderi *et al.* (1997)	Children	Outpatient strabismus	Prevention R, DB, PC** (metoclopramide, ondansetron)	5
Goodarzi (1998)	Children (2-14 years)	Major orthopaedic	Prevention R, DB, PC** (ondansetron)	40

R = randomised; DB = double blind; PC = placebo controlled; * = no difference to placebo; ** = significant difference to placebo

Table 3.5 Overall impression of droperidol

Benefits	*Drawbacks*
Widely used by anaesthetists	Variable efficacy
Reasonable efficacy for prevention	Many reports of side-effects
Considered a 'standard' for other drugs	Onset of side-effects may be delayed
	Little evidence of 'treatment' effect

Phenothiazines

Phenothiazines were originally developed in the late 19th century by chemists working in the dye industry. Later, promethazine was found to have profound hypnotic properties and from that compound the anti-emetic drugs, prochlorperazine and perphenazine were developed. In his review, Rowbotham (1992) observed that although prochlorperazine had been in clinical use since the 1950s for the prevention of PONV, there had been precious few studies and certainly no modern randomised controlled studies with which to evaluate its efficacy. Although widely used in clinical practice in both prophylactic and treatment roles, it is only licensed for the latter indication and then only as a single dose.

To much the same extent, very little is known about perphenazine, although favoured by many older anaesthetists as part of the 'recipe' for patients at high risk of PONV. However, a recent study (Steinbrook *et al.* 1998) has shown perphenazine to be as effective as combinations of ondansetron plus droperidol, and metoclopramide plus droperidol.

Side-effects. The major perceived side-effect of phenothiazine is extrapyramidal reaction, though the evidence for it being any worse than other dopaminergic agents is scanty. However, Robbie (1959) suggested that such reactions were more likely after perphenazine than prochlorperazine. As both drugs have sedative qualities, it is hardly surprising that they may cause delays in recovery from anaesthesia.

The overall impression of phenothiazines in clinical practice is shown in Table 3.6.

Anticholinergics

The only anticholinergic that has been shown to have anti-emetic qualities is hyoscine. However, there have been very few studies on hyoscine used for PONV, with most of the literature dating back to before 1990. If administered intravenously, hyoscine can cause confusion and delayed recovery from anaesthesia. Although used primarily for its 'drying' effects, the papaveretum/hyoscine ('om and scop') pre-medication may have some anti-emetic benefits. Even so, dry mouth is a commom complaint of patients given hyoscine. In the management of motion sickness, transdermal hyoscine has been shown to be useful but when used for PONV, the patch has to be applied well in advance of the precipitary factors.

Table 3.6 Overall impression of phenothiazines

Benefits	*Drawbacks*
Widely used by ward staff	Variable efficacy
Perphenazine recently shown to be as effective as ondansetron (Steinbrook *et al.* 1998)	Many reports of side-effects
	Very few controlled studies
	Only licensed for treatment

Overall, there is a feeling, though good clinical studies have not been performed, that hyoscine may be a useful drug in patients where the chief stimulus to PONV is of a vestibular origin.

Antihistaminics

Drugs of several types (e.g. piperazines, phenothiazines) exhibit histamine type-1 receptor antagonist activity and many are anti-emetics. While many antihistamines have been used in the management of motion sickness, only cyclizine has been developed for the treatment of PONV.

Cyclizine

Cyclizine is a piperazine derivative and has antimuscarinic, in addition to antihistaminic, actions. The main body of studies of cyclizine dates back to the 1960s and very few have been undertaken since then. However, cyclizine has grown in popularity for the treatment of PONV where, anecdotally, it seems to be as good as any other agent. Watts (1996) showed a rather disappointing incidence of PONV in day-cases of 51 per cent with cyclizine which was comparable to that achieved in a pilot study when no anti-emetic therapy was given. Cyclizine has also been given in combination with PCA morphine (Walder & Aitkenhead 1995). In this study, the incidence of PONV with cyclizine was 28 per cent.

On the positive side, cyclizine seems to have few major side-effects, in particular, there are no extrapyramidal side-effects. Sedation and a dry mouth are often present; a consequence of the antimuscarinic activity.

Cyclizine, for no real scientific reasons, does appear to have developed a niche in the treatment of PONV.

An anti-emetic effect is only associated with H_1 receptor antagonists. A study with the H_2 receptor blocker, ranitidine, showed no difference to placebo (Cozanitis *et al.* 1996).

Antiserotonergic drugs – 5-HT_3 antagonists

This group of drugs has evolved from the development of anti-emetics for use in chemotherapy, particularly cisplatin. The observation that high-dose metoclopramide was partially effective in the prevention of cisplatin-induced nausea and vomiting led to the discovery that the 5-HT_3 receptor was involved in the process. There can be little denying that these drugs have had a dramatic effect on chemotherapy-induced nausea and vomiting. However, the introduction of 5-HT_3 antagonists into practice for the prevention and treatment of PONV has not been so successful, possibly as a consequence of the limited involvement of 5-HT_3 release in the PONV process.

Ondansetron

Ondansetron is probably the best investigated of the 5-HT_3 antagonists. A number of studies have been undertaken on ondansetron, both compared with placebo and, more lately, active anti-emetics. A summary of recent randomised, controlled studies on ondansetron is shown in Table 3.7. Three of the studies were placebo-controlled and showed a difference to placebo. A fourth placebo-controlled study by Maestre *et al.* (1997) had such a low incidence of PONV for all groups that comparison is difficult. In comparison with other agents, ondansetron has shown superior efficacy in its preventive role (Diemunsch *et al.* 1997a). In two paediatric studies (Scuderi *et al.* 1997; Goodarzi 1998), ondansetron was shown to be superior to placebo and, in the latter, to droperidol.

Granisetron

Granisetron has similar properties to ondansetron and has been investigated in a number of settings by predominantly one group. A summary of the studies is shown in Table 3.8. In all studies containing a placebo control group there was a significant difference with granisetron.

Dolasetron

Dolasetron has recently been introduced to the US market and is, in many respects, very similar to the other 5-HT_3 antagonists. To date the majority of literature relates to dose-ranging, placebo-controlled studies and so it is difficult to make a fair comparison to the other 'setrons'. Recent studies are summarised in Table 3.9.

Tropisetron

Tropisetron has very similar properties and has conflictingly been shown to have less effect than ondansetron and granisetron (Nagiub *et al.* 1996) and more effect than ondansetron (Pascucci *et al.* 1996).

Table 3.7 Summary of recent studies on ondansetron

Reference	*Type of patient*	*Type of surgery*	*Type of study (comparators)*	*Incidence of PONV (%)*
Maestre *et al.* (1997)	Adults	Ambulatory	Prevention R, DB, PC* (metoclopramide, droperidol)	6
Gan *et al.* (1994)	Adults	Hip and knee replacement	Prevention R, DB, PC** (droperidol)	17
Watts (1996)	Adult females	Laparoscopic surgery	Prevention R, DB (cyclizine, metoclopramide)	20
Nagiub *et al.* (1996)	Adults	Laparoscopic cholecystectomy	Prevention R, DB, PC** (tropisetron, granisetron, metoclopramide)	34
Sung *et al.* (1993)	Adult females	Ambulatory gynaecology	Prevention R, DB, PC** (no active comparator)	38
Diemunsch *et al.* (1997a)	Adults	General surgery	Treatment R, DB (metoclopramide)	41
Scuderi *et al.* (1997)	Children	Outpatient strabismus	Prevention R, DB, PC** (metoclopramide, droperidol)	5
Goodarzi (1998)	Children (2–14 years)	Major orthopaedic	Prevention R, DB, PC** (droperidol)	25

R = randomised; DB = double blind; PC = placebo controlled; * = no difference to placebo; ** = significant difference to placebo

Table 3.8 Summary of recent studies on granisetron

Reference	*Type of patient*	*Type of surgery*	*Type of study (comparators)*	*Incidence of PONV (%)*
Fujii *et al.* (1998b)	Adult females	Thyroid surgery	Prevention R, DB, PC** (with 100 μg/kg)* (with 20 μg/kg) (three doses of granisetron)	12 (100 μg/kg) 56 (20 μg/kg)
Fujii *et al.* (1998d)	Adults	Middle ear surgery	Prevention R, DB (droperidol, metoclopramide)	15
Fujii *et al.* (1998c)	Adult females	Breast surgery	Prevention R, DB, PC** (droperidol, metoclopramide)	17
Fujii *et al.* (1998a)	Adult females with history of PONV	Major gynaecology	Prevention R, DB (droperidol, metoclopramide)	20
Fujii *et al.* (1997)	Adult females with history of motion sickness	Major gynaecology	Prevention R, DB, PC** (droperidol, metoclopramide)	23
Nagiub *et al.* (1996)	Adults	Laparoscopic cholecystectomy	Prevention R,DB, PC** (tropisetron, ondansetron, metoclopramide)	48

R = randomised; DB = double blind; PC = placebo controlled; * = no difference to placebo; ** = significant difference to placebo

Table 3.9 Summary of recent studies on dolasetron

Reference	*Type of patient*	*Type of surgery*	*Type of study (comparators)*	*Incidence of PONV (%)*
Kortilla *et al.* (1997)	Adults	Range of surgery	Prevention R, DB, PC** (ondansetron)	29 (50 mg)
Diemunsch *et al.* (1997b)	Adult females	Gynaecology	Prevention R, DB, PC** (different doses of dolasetron)	33 (25 mg)
Graczyk *et al.* (1997)	Adult females	Laparoscopy	Prevention R, DB, PC** (different doses of dolasetron)	44 (50 mg)
Warriner *et al.* (1997)	Adult females	Abdominal hysterectomy	Prevention O, R, DB, PC** (different doses of dolasetron)	46 (100 mg)
Diemunsch *et al.* (1997c)	Adults	Range of surgery	Treatment R, DB, PC** (different doses of dolasetron)	62 (50 mg)
Kovac *et al.* (1997)	Adults	Outpatient	Treatment R, DB, PC** (different doses of dolasetron)	65 (12.5 mg)

O = oral; R = randomised; DB = double blind; PC = placebo controlled; * = no difference to placebo; ** = significant difference to placebo

Other 'setrons'

Other setrons, such as lerisetron and alosetron, are currently under investigation for chemotherapy-induced nausea and vomiting and may, in time, find their way into PONV practice.

Side-effects of 5-HT$_3$ antagonists

These are very rare, being restricted largely to headache. There is no evidence of extrapyramidal reactions. Recently, there has been some concern regarding the risk of QT changes in the electrocardiograph associated with dolasetron which could lead to arrhythmias; however, it is unclear if this has any implications for the other drugs in the group. Overall, these drugs are considered to be safe.

The overall impression of the 5-HT$_3$ drugs is shown in Table 3.10.

Neurokinin-1 (NK$_1$) receptor antagonists

These are the latest generation of drugs undergoing investigation. They appear to act by preventing the vomiting process rather than blocking the afferent input. In animal studies, these drugs appear able to prevent vomiting from any cause, but whether they are effective in preventing nausea remains unclear. Early human studies show promise that this effectiveness in animal work will be translated into humans.

Other treatments

Propofol

Propofol, given in low doses, has been said to reduce the incidence of PONV. However, two studies – one by Lacroix (1996) looking at the treatment of established PONV, the other by Montgomery *et al.* (1996) in the prevention of PONV – have been unable to show an effect.

Cannabinoids

Cannabinoids have been suggested as effective anti-emetics. Most reports are anecdotal, with the only comparison showing nabilone to be less effective than metoclopramide (Lewis *et al.* 1994).

PONV management options

Prevention

In considering the prevention options, the 5-HT$_3$ receptor antagonists appear to be the best option, with the highest efficacy of the currently available drugs. This impression is further enhanced when their very limited side-effect profile is taken into account.

Table 3.10 Overall impression of 5-HT_3 receptor blockers

Benefits	*Drawbacks*
Shown to be highly effective in chemotherapy	? effective against opioid-induced nausea and vomiting
Very low incidence of side-effects	Expensive
Most effective of the currently available agents for both prevention and treatment	? problems with QTc and arrhythmias

Treatment

There have been very few studies looking at treatment. Cyclizine and prochlorperazine are widely used but the only comparative study (Diemunsch 1997a) shows a benefit of ondansetron over metoclopramide, although dolasetron has been shown to be more effective than placebo. That coupled with the setrons' side-effect profile suggests them to be reasonable drugs for this purpose.

To treat or to prevent?

There must remain a dilemma as to whether one should try to prevent PONV or treat it as and when it occurs. One factor that must be taken into account is the balance between efficacy of prevention and the incidence of side-effects. If one uses a philosophy of the 'number needed to treat' to prevent one episode of PONV, one can have a measure of efficacy but often the incidence of side-effects of the drugs is not so clear. In a study on PONV after squint surgery, Tramer *et al.* (1991) could show a definite efficacy:side-effect ratio for ondansetron. Figures for other drugs or indications may not be so convincing.

Conclusions

Despite the wide range of anti-emetic agents, one is still left with the knowledge that:

- no single agent is 100 per cent effective in all cases;
- no drug is completely free of side-effects, although for some agents such side-effects are minimal;
- newer anti-emetic agents are relatively expensive;
- it may be unreasonable to administer a drug to a large number of patients in order to prevent PONV in only a few.

It can only be hoped that the next generation of anti-emetics will help to solve this problem. In the meantime, the best approach may be the use of combination therapy.

References

Bateman DN, Rawlins MD & Simpson JM (1965). Extrapyramidal reactions to metoclopramide. *British Medical Journal* **291**, 930–2.

Caldwell C, Rains G & McKiterick K (1987). An unusual reaction to preoperative metoclopramide. *Anesthesiology* **67**, 854–5.

Cozanitis D, Asantila R, Eklund P *et al.* (1996). A comparison of ranitidine, droperidol or placebo in the prevention of nausea and vomiting after hysterectomy. *Canadian Journal of Anaesthesia* **43**, 106–9.

Diemunsch P, Conseiller C, Clyti N *et al.* (1997a). Ondansetron compared with metoclopramide in the treatment of established postoperative nausea and vomiting. *British Journal of Anaesthesia* **79**, 322–6.

Diemunsch P, D'Hollander A, Paxton L *et al.* (1997b). Intravenous dolasetron mesilate in the prevention of postoperative nausea and vomiting in females undergoing gynecological surgery. *Journal of Clinical Anesthesia* **9**, 365–73.

Diemunsch P, Leeser J, Feiss P *et al.* (1997c). Intravenous dolasetron mesilate ameliorates postoperative nausea and vomiting. *Canadian Journal of Anaesthesia* **44**, 173–81.

Dundee JW & Clarke RSJ (1973). The premedicant and anti-emetic action of metoclopramide. *Postgraduate Medical Journal* **49**(Suppl.4), 34–8.

Ellis FR & Spence AA (1970). Clinical trials of metoclopramide (Maxolon) as an antiemetic in anaesthesia. *Anaesthesia* **25**, 368–71.

Foster PN, Stickle BR & Laurence AS (1996). Akathisia following low-dose droperidol for antiemesis in day-case patients. *Anaesthesia* **51**, 491–4.

Fujii Y, Toyooka H & Tanaka H (1997). Prevention of PONV with granisetron, droperidol and metoclopramide in female patients with history of motion sickness. *Canadian Journal of Anaesthesia* **44**, 820–4.

Fujii Y, Saitoh Y, Tanaka H *et al.* (1998a). Prevention of PONV with granisetron, droperidol or metoclopramide in patients with postoperative emesis. *Canadian Journal of Anaesthesia* **45**, 153–6.

Fujii Y, Saitoh Y, Tanaka H *et al.* (1998b). Prophylactic antiemetic therapy with granisetron in women undergoing thyroidectomy. *British Journal of Anaesthesia* **81**, 526–8.

Fujii Y, Tanaka H & Toyooka H (1998c). Prevention of nausea and vomiting in female patients undergoing breast surgery: a comparison with granisetron, droperidol, metoclopramide and placebo. *Acta Anaesthesiologica Scandinavica* **42**, 220–4.

Fujii Y, Toyooka H & Tanaka H (1998d). Prophylactic anti-emetic therapy with granisetron, droperidol and metoclopramide in female patients undergoing middle ear surgery. *Anaesthesia* **53**, 1165–8.

Gan TJ, Collis R & Hetreed M (1994). Double-blind comparison of ondansetron, droperidol and saline in the prevention of postoperative nausea and vomiting. *British Journal of Anaesthesia* **72**, 544–7.

Goodarzi M (1998). A double blind comparison of droperidol and ondansetron for prevention of emesis in children undergoing orthopaedic surgery. *Paediatric Anaesthesia* **8**, 325–9.

Graczyk SG, McKenzie R, Kaller S *et al.* (1997). Intravenous dolasetron for the prevention of postoperative nausea and vomiting after outpatient laparoscopic gynecologic surgery. *Anesthesia and Analgesia* **84**, 325–30.

Harrington RA, Hamilton CW, Brogden RN *et al.* (1983). Metoclopramide: an updated review of its pharmacological properties and clinical use. *Drugs* **25**, 451–94.

Judkins KC & Harmer M (1982). Haloperidol as an adjunct analgesic in the management of postoperative pain. *Anaesthesia* **37**, 1118–20.

Kortilla K, Clergue F, Leeser J *et al.* (1997). Intravenous dolasetron and ondansetron in the prevention of postoperative nausea and vomiting: a multicenter, double-blind, placebo-controlled study. *Acta Anaesthesiologica Scandinavica* **41**, 914–22.

Kovac AL, Scuderi PE, Boerner TF *et al.* (1997). Treatment of postoperative nausea and vomiting with single intravenous doses of dolasetron mesylate, a multicenter trial. *Anesthesia and Analgesia* **85**, 546–52.

Lacroix G, Lessard MR & Trepanier CA (1996). Treatment of post-operative nausea and vomiting: comparison of propofol, droperidol and metoclopramide. *Canadian Journal of Anaesthesia* **43**, 115–20.

Lamond CT, Robinson DL, Boyd JD *et al.* (1998). Addition of droperidol to morphine administered by the patient-controlled analgesia method: what is the optimal dose? *European Journal of Anaesthesiology* **15**, 304–9.

Lewis IH, Campbell DN & Barrowcliffe MP (1994). Effect of nabilone on nausea and vomiting after total abdominal hysterectomy. *British Journal of Anaesthesia* **73**, 244–6.

Loo CC, Thomas E, Tan HM *et al.* (1997). A comparison of the antiemetic efficacy of droperidol alone and in combination with metoclopramide in day surgery anaesthesia. *Medical Journal of Malaysia* **52**, 264–8.

Maestre JM, Puente J & Dierssen T (1997). Prevention of postoperative nausea and vomiting with metoclopramide, droperidol and ondansetron: a randomized, double-blind comparison with placebo in ambulatory surgery. *Ambulatory Surgery* **5**, 153–9.

Montgomery JE, Sutherland CJ, Kestin IG *et al.* (1996). Infusions of subhypnotic doses of propofol for the prevention of postoperative nausea and vomiting. *Anaesthesia* **51**, 554–7.

Nagiub M, El Bakry AK, Kloshim MHB *et al.* (1996). Prophylactic antiemetic therapy with ondansetron, tropisetron, granisetron and metoclopramide in patients undergoing laparoscopic cholecystectomy: a randomized, double-blind comparison with placebo. *Canadian Journal of Anaesthesia* **43**, 226–31.

Pascucci G, Palmieri V, Miranda G *et al.* (1996). Tropisetron versus ondansetron in the prevention and control of postoperative nausea and vomiting. *Acta Anaesthesiologica Italica* **47**, 173–7.

Pegg MS (1980). Hypotension following metoclopramide injection. *Anaesthesia* **35**, 614–6.

Robbie DS (1959). Postanaesthetic vomiting and anti-emetic drugs. *Anaesthesia* **14**, 349–54.

Rowbotham DJ (1992). Current management of postoperative nausea and vomiting. *British Journal of Anaesthesia* **69**(Suppl.1), 46S–59S.

Scuderi PE, Weaver RG Jr, James RL *et al.* (1997). A randomized double-blind, placebo controlled comparison of droperidol, ondansetron, and metoclopramide for the prevention of vomiting following outpatient strabismus surgery in children. *Journal of the Clinical Anesthesia* **9**, 551–8.

Steinbrook RA, Gosnell JL & Freiberger D (1998). Prophylactic antiemetics for laparoscopic cholecystectomy: a comparison of perphenazine, droperidol plus ondansetron, and droperidol plus metoclopramide. *Journal of Clinical Anesthesia* **10**, 494–8.

Stienstra R, Samhan YM, El-Mofty M *et al.* (1997). Double-blind comparison of alizapride, droperidol and ondansetron in the treatment of post-operative nausea. *European Journal of Anaesthesiology* **14**, 290–4.

Sung Y-F, Wetchler BV, Duncalf D *et al.* (1993). A double-blind, placebo controlled pilot study examining the effectiveness of intravenous ondansetron in the prevention of postoperative nausea and emesis. *Journal of Clinical Anesthesia* **5**, 22–9.

Thorpe J & Smith AF (1996). A case of postoperative anxiety due to low dose droperidol used with patient-controlled analgesia. *International Journal of Obstetric Anesthesia* **5**, 283–4.

Tramer M, Moore A & McQuay H (1995). Prevention of vomiting after paediatric strabismus surgery: a systematic review using the number-needed-to-treat method. *British Journal of Anaesthesia* **75**, 556–61.

Walder AD & Aitkenhead AR (1995). A comparison of droperidol and cyclizine in the prevention of postoperative nausea and vomiting associated with patient-controlled analgesia. *Anaesthesia* **50**, 654–6.

Warriner CB, Knox D, Belo S *et al.* (1997). Prophylactic oral dolasetron mesylate reduces nausea and vomiting after abdominal hysterectomy. *Canadian Journal of Anaesthesia* **44**, 1167–73.

Watts SA (1996). A randomized double-blinded comparison of metoclopramide, ondansetron and cyclizine in day-case laparoscopy. *Anaesthesia and Intensive Care* **24**, 546–51.

Chapter 4

Evidentiary basis of non-pharmacological interventions in PONV

Karen H Simpson

Introduction

PONV is a still major problem (Rowbotham 1992). Several non-pharmacological approaches have been used to treat emesis after surgery, including:

- manoeuvres which affect peri-operative stomach contents;
- psychological techniques such as suggestion or hypnosis;
- acupuncture techniques;
- use of plant derivatives.

These approaches are examined below.

Peri-operative stomach contents

The duration of peri-operative fasting may influence PONV. It has been suggested that depriving patients of oral fluids before surgery may increase PONV. In patients undergoing early termination of pregnancy under propofol and alfentanil anaesthesia, administration of 150 ml clear fluid 1.5–2.0 hours prior to surgery did not alter the incidence of PONV (Goodwin *et al.* 1991). However, the incidence of PONV was low overall, so this finding should be interpreted with caution. A study of 100 similar patients assessed the effect of administration of 1,000 ml clear fluid intravenously during propofol and alfentanil anaesthesia (Elhakim *et al.* 1998). Nausea scores were significantly lower in the fluid-treated group during the 24–48 hours after surgery. The incidence of emesis was lower in the fluid-treated group, as was the time to tolerate oral fluids. Intra-operative fluid administration may therefore protect this group against PONV.

Factors such as a large residual gastric volume or manual ventilation with a bag and mask (leading to gases distending the stomach) may influence the incidence of PONV. A study of 265 day-patients concluded that aspiration of gastric contents with an orogastric tube did not influence the incidence of PONV within 24 hours after surgery (Trepanier & Isabel 1993). A study of 201 patients having hysterectomy also showed that gastric aspiration did not affect PONV (Hovorjka *et al.* 1990). Gastric aspiration may actually have led to increased PONV. A study of 189 patients having hysterectomy concluded that the experience of the anaesthetist who was ventilating the patient's lungs affected the incidence of PONV (Hovorjka *et al.* 1990). More junior staff had a higher rate of PONV for up to 6 hours after surgery.

Early administration of oral fluid may increase PONV, particularly in children. A study of 317 children undergoing day-surgery involved either administering fluids ad lib or withholding oral fluids for 4–6 hours after surgery (Kearney 1998). All children received intravenous fluids to cover the period of fasting. Those who had fluids withheld had significantly less vomiting in the first day after surgery (38 per cent) compared with those who drank ad lib (56 per cent). The difference was most apparent in children who received opioids.

Attention to factors affecting the contents of the stomach in the peri-operative period may be an important part of the management of PONV. Further research in this area is needed.

Psychological techniques

It may be possible to influence patients' post-operative state after surgery by using psychological techniques before, during or after surgery. Pre-operative preparation of patients using hypnosis and relaxation via audiotapes has been used to try to reduce PONV (Enqvist *et al.* 1997). Fifty women scheduled for breast reduction were randomised to either no intervention or listening to an audiotape for 4–6 days prior to surgery. The tape used hypnotic induction followed by guided relaxation to states incompatible with emesis. Patients in the hypnosis group had significantly less nausea and vomited less than controls (39 versus 68 per cent).

Pre-operative positive suggestion was assessed in a study of 226 patients (Lauder *et al.* 1995). Patients in the positive-suggestion group were told that the incidence of PONV was to be greatly reduced by the use of two anti-emetic drugs. Patients in the control group were simply told that they were in a study of post-operative well-being, with no reference to PONV. Nausea, vomiting or retching was the same in both groups, but the use of anti-emetics was reduced in the suggestion group. This is difficult to interpret. The suggestion group may have felt that they had already received powerful anti-emetics and there was no value in accepting more.

There is evidence that therapeutic suggestions given during light sedation or anaesthesia can produce effects on the patient (Evans & Richardson 1988). In a study of 39 patients having hysterectomy, 19 were played a tape of positive therapeutic suggestions and 20 were played a blank tape during surgery. Those in the suggestion group spent less time in hospital, suffered a shorter period of pyrexia after surgery and were generally rated by nurses as having a better than expected recovery. Sixty women undergoing gynaecological surgery were randomised to receive positive suggestions or no intervention (Williams *et al.* 1994). Those who received positive suggestion had significantly less PONV in the first day after surgery. Fifty women having abdominal hysterectomy were randomised to hear either positive suggestions or a blank tape via headphones during anaesthesia (Maroof *et al.* 1997). In those who listened to suggestion, vomiting was reduced (36 versus 60 per cent) and the use of anti-emetic was less (22 versus 67 per cent).

One hundred patients undergoing thyroidectomy under neurolept anaesthesia were randomised to hear either positive non-affirmative suggestions during the whole of anaesthesia or a blank tape (Eberhart *et al.* 1998). The suggestion group had significantly less PONV (47 versus 86 per cent) and required less anti-emetic (31 versus 69 per cent). The use of hypnosis as an adjunct to local anaesthesia with conscious intravenous sedation was studied in 337 patients undergoing major and minor plastic surgery (Faymonville *et al.* 1995). Midazolam and alfentanil alone were used in 172 patients, hypnosis to trance level was used in 172 patients and relaxation was used in 28 patients. In all three groups midazolam and alfentanil were titrated to achieve patient comfort and immobility. PONV was reported in 1 per cent of hypnosis patients compared with 13 per cent in the relaxation group and 27 per cent in the sedation-only group. The hypnosis group had lower pain scores and required less alfentanil, therefore the reduction in emesis may have been due to opioid sparing.

Some studies have failed to demonstrate an effect for psychological intervention. Seventy-five patients having hysterectomy were allocated to listen either to one of three tapes containing positive therapeutic suggestion on to a blank tape (Lui *et al.* 1992). No effect was demonstrated. Seventy females having breast surgery were randomised to listen to a message with reassuring information focused on reducing PONV during anaesthesia, the other group were played a blank tape (Oddby-Muhrbeck *et al.* 1995). No difference in PONV was detected within the first 24 hours. However, those who heard the suggestion tape had a lower recall of nausea and vomiting. Therefore it was suggested that some implicit processing after therapeutic suggestion may have occurred.

Psychological techniques may have a place in the management of PONV. Trial design, method of delivery of suggestion, timing of suggestion, type of anaesthesia and surgery may have an influence on the effect of this type of intervention. Individual patient factors may also play an important role.

Acupuncture techniques

References to the use of acupuncture began to appear in the English medical literature about 150 years ago (Saks 1991). Interest declined over the early part of the last century and has re-emerged in the past 30 years. Acupuncture is popular again. A survey in 1995 assessed 8,745 people and found that one in four used complementary medicine, of whom 12 per cent used acupuncture. This compares with a similar survey in 1986 which showed 1 in 12 people were using complementary therapy (Anon 1995).

Complementary therapies need to be examined carefully. Clinical effectiveness has not been demonstrated, in ways which can be considered as conclusive, for the use of acupuncture in many areas of medicine. Purchasers of health care have an ethical obligation to use resources for the greatest good. They need accurate and reliable estimates of the cost benefits of complementary techniques as well as evidence of efficacy and safety. Patients must be protected from useless treatments. Effective, safe and cheap therapies should be identified so that they can be integrated into conventional medicine. Researchers need to be aware that clinical trials of acupuncture need a different set of methodological assumptions from drug trials. At present, research methods in acupuncture still need to meet all conventional methodological requirements.

There are obstacles to rigorous acupuncture research and studies of acupuncture often score quite low for methodological quality (ter Reit *et al.* 1990). There are some unique difficulties when trying to design good acupuncture trials. Acupuncture research is often done by enthusiasts, which may lead to bias. There are many different forms of acupuncture treatment – it is not just one simple therapy.

Acupuncture, acupressure, electrical stimulation, injection and the use of lasers on the whole body or sometimes in confined areas, such as the ear, are all used. These treatments may not be directly comparable and so interpretation can be difficult. The diagnosis used to plan treatment is not always traditional. Each patient is treated as unique. Diagnoses which do not seem scientifically valid are used to make treatment plans. Therapy is often not standardised. Each patient may be treated differently and individuals may have different treatments on different occasions. Acupuncture by formula is not ideal and is different from the traditional method of treatment. Failure to demonstrate efficacy of acupuncture performed using a standard recipe for all patients is not equivalent to showing ineffectiveness of traditional acupuncture. The other variable is of course the skill of the therapist. Acupuncture points are of varying size and depth. Points can also vary within the individual depending on whether they are healthy or not. There are many schools of thought about acupuncture points. However, most acupuncturists are in agreement that it is necessary to produce 'needling sensation' during treatment. Blinding during acupuncture trials is difficult. Patients in non-acupuncture groups must believe that they are having an effective treatment. It is possible that in some individuals, who are very sensitive to acupuncture, any point can produce an effect, if stimulated. Therefore the treatment of so called 'sham' points may not be the same as no treatment at all. Blinding of the operator is not possible, observations must be done by an independent observer. The use of a placebo treatment is one of the most difficult issues in acupuncture research. The use of a placebo group in research is only ethical if uncertainty exists about the best treatment for an individual and if there is no evidence that one treatment is more effective than another. The use of a placebo in acupuncture research in PONV is not ethical (Adams 1996). When using electrical acupuncture it may be easier to provide a placebo by either using subthreshold stimulation or not passing electrical current in the placebo group.

A survey of clinical trials of acupuncture collected 228 trials, 137 were on pain and 21 were on emesis (Kaptchuk *et al.* 1996). Many of the studies of chronic pain were too contradictory to reach a consensus. Considering all the potential difficulties with acupuncture research it would appear that studying the use of the technique in the treatment of PONV may be valuable. Many of the difficulties with acupuncture trials can be reduced when studying emesis. Nausea and vomiting are more simple to treat using acupuncture than many other conditions: they can be managed using a single point which is often the same for different individuals; there is a short follow-up time when dealing with PONV; and there is a reproducible endpoint with objective outcome measures.

A systematic review examined acupuncture trials for the management of emesis worldwide until March 1995 (Vickers 1996). Forty-two trials were found on the use of P6 stimulation for PONV, cancer therapy or pregnancy-related emesis. Papers were ranked after assessment of their methodological robustness. Nine papers were excluded after assessment (all of which favoured acupuncture). The method of P6 stimulation varied:

Manual or electrical	11
Manual acupressure	4
Wrist bands	2
TENS	2
Injection	2

The use of controls varied:

None	9
Historical	1
Acupuncture under general anaesthesia	5
Acupuncture with local anaesthesia	1
Dummy points	1
Placebo wrist bands	2
Sham TENS	2

Four trials of P6 acupuncture under general anaesthesia showed no effect. Twenty-seven of the remaining 29 studies showed an effect with acupuncture. There were only 12 randomised placebo-controlled trials of P6 acupuncture not under general anaesthesia; 11 of the 12 showed an effect for acupuncture. Eight of the randomised placebo controlled trials concerned PONV (see Box 4.1).

The review showed that seven different centres had used different methods to stimulate P6 in adults and children of different sexes. A further study in 1994 which involved 46 women having gynaecological surgery was not included in the review (Allen *et al.* 1994). Those who had P6 stimulation rather than sham treatment had no difference in PONV, but had a reduced requirement for anti-emetics. A literature

Box 4.1

- P6 acupuncture versus dummy acupuncture versus no treatment, n=75 females, minor gynaecological surgery, number of patients symptom-free after surgery = acupuncture 76%, dummy acupuncture 24%, controls 24% (P<0.001) (Dundee *et al.* 1986)
- P6 acupuncture versus no treatment, n=500 males and females, general surgery, incidence of vomiting = acupuncture 4.4%, controls 16% (P<0.001) (Fry 1986)
- Wrist bands versus dummy wrist bands versus prochlorperazine, n=152 males and females, general surgery, nausea days 1 and 2 = wrist bands less than dummy bands and prochlorperazine (P<0.02), nausea days 3–6 = no difference (Barsoum *et al.* 1990)
- P6 acupuncture after injection of local anaesthetic versus P6 acupuncture after injection of saline, n=74 females, minor gynaecological surgery, symptom-free within 6 hours of surgery = local anaesthesia 52%, saline 81% (P<0.013) (Dundee & Ghaly 1991)
- Wrist bands versus dummy wrist bands, n=66 male and female children, squint surgery, number vomiting within 24 hours = wrist bands 92%, controls 83%, not significant (Lewis *et al.* 1991)
- P6 acupressure versus dummy acupressure versus no treatment, n=90 females, minor gynaecological surgery = P6 acupressure better than dummy acupressure or no treatment for nausea within first 6 hours after surgery (Gieron *et al.* 1993)
- P6 TENS stimulation versus sham P6 TENS, n=103 females after hysterectomy = TENS better than sham TENS for control of vomiting during 36 hours after surgery (Fassoulaki *et al.* 1993)
- P6 TENS full stimulation versus P6 TENS subthreshold stimulation versus P6 sham TENS versus no treatment, n=230 males and females, orthopaedic surgery = TENS full stimulation reduced sickness severity in females only (P<0.001) (McMillan 1994)

search covering the period March 1995–December 1998 revealed ten more trials on the use of P6 stimulation for PONV. Three studies had methodological problems and one study was designed to look at post-operative pain and any change in emesis was incidental (see Box 4.2).

Previous systematic reviews of acupuncture have often given equivocal findings. A review of acupuncture in chronic pain showed that only 11 of 51 studies were good enough for inclusion (ter Reit *et al.* 1990). P6 acupuncture is easier to study. Overall the evidence for its efficacy in the treatment of PONV is good. A psychological cause for its efficacy is unlikely. Dummy points and dummy wrist bands are less effective than real stimulation. The difference between true points and dummy points cannot be explained by patient belief. It is important to remember that much of the work has been done in adult females: only 22 per cent of subjects in the 14 randomised controlled trials were male (Figure 4.1). There is an obvious difference if acupuncture is performed under general anaesthesia, the timing of opioid medication may have an influence (Dundee & Ghaly 1989). Local anaesthesia blocks the effect of acupuncture.

Box 4.2

- P6 wrist bands versus placebo, n=60, post-Caesarean section under regional block with spinal opioid, P6 wrist bands emesis reduced for 48 hours (Ho *et al.* 1996)
- Transcutaneous stimulation of P6 and LI4 versus no treatment administered after anaesthesia, n=84 children, no significant difference between groups (Schwager *et al.* 1996)
- P6 wrist bands versus dummy wrist bands, n=200, short surgery, incidence of emesis P6 group 23% and dummy group 41% (P<0.0058) (Fan *et al.* 1997)
- P6 stimulation after anaesthesia but before opioid treatment versus no stimulation, n=81, minor gynaecological day case surgery, P6 group decreased PONV for 24 hours after surgery. Acupuncture helped a subset of patients with a prior history of PONV and motion sickness. Placebo group had 16 times risk of PONV, while in hospital and 4 times risk in 24 hours after discharge, 3 of placebo group had to be admitted to hospital because of emesis (Al-Sadi *et al.* 1997)
- P6 wrist bands versus metoclopramide versus placebo, n=75 patients after Caesarean section, P6 wrist bands and metoclopramide reduced emesis compared with placebo (Stein *et al.* 1997)
- P6 stimulation by laser versus placebo, n=40 children after strabismus surgery, vomiting within 24 hours = P6 25%, placebo (85%) (P<0.0001) (Schlager *et al.* 1998)

Vicker's systematic review

Total patients n = 2,045 (all 21 PONV studies included)

Adults n = 1,845	Males	299 (16%)
	Females	1,545 (84%)
Children n = 201 (10%)		

Randomised controlled trials only

Total patients n = 1,580 (14 trials) (Boxes 4.1 & 4.2)

Adults n = 1,390	Males	310 (22%)
	Females	1,080 (78%)
Children n = 190 (12%)		

Sources: Vickers (1996) & literature searches (1995–8)

Figure 4.1 Summary of patients involved in studies discussed

It is important to accurately localise acupuncture points if treatment is to be effective. The mode of stimulus is probably not important as long as the stimulus is in the correct place. Treatment should ideally be given prior to the emetic stimulus. Duration of P6 effect may be about 6 hours, as suggested by study in patients having chemotherapy

(Dundee & Young 1990). The effect may be prolonged by applying acupressure over P6 every 2 hours. Four studies of children have been described, only the one which used laser showed an effect. One trial involved stimulation under anaesthesia, so that the negative result was not surprising. Children are often very sensitive to acupuncture so the lack of efficacy in this group is difficult to explain. Only 12 per cent subjects studied in the 14 randomised controlled trials reported were children. Strong stimulation during acupuncture can produce the problem it is being used to treat, called aggravation. Perhaps stimulation was too strong for these children, especially in the group where P6 and LI4 were stimulated.

The use of plant derivatives such as ginger and mint

These will not be considered in detail as they are strictly pharmacological, although unconventional. The powdered rhizome of *Zingiber officinale* (the common ginger root) is a traditional treatment for gastrointestinal complaints dating from the ninth century, being regarded as a carmitive and spasmolytic agent. The active ingredient in ginger root and its mechanism of action are unknown. A local effect on the gut has been proposed. It has been used to treat motion sickness and vertigo. It can reduce cisplatin-induced emesis and delayed gastric emptying in animals (Sharma & Gupta 1998). It can be used to treat hyperemesis gravidarum (Fischer-Rasmussen *et al.* 1991). Some studies have demonstrated that oral pre-medication with ginger is as successful as metoclopramide for PONV (Bone *et al.* 1990; Phillips *et al.* 1993). However, its efficacy in the treatment of PONV is unproven (Arfen *et al.* 1995; Visalyaputra *et al.* 1998). One study of the use of peppermint oil for post-operative nausea, in a small group of patients having gynaecological surgery, suggested that it may be efficacious (Tate 1997), but more rigorous study is needed.

Conclusions

Non-pharmacological methods may be useful in the management of PONV. They often have advantages, such as ease of use, safety and low cost. Such methods must be rigorously assessed. Only those treatments which can be shown to be of value should be adopted into current practice. The use of a method just because it seems innocuous should be discouraged, unless its efficacy can be shown. A scientific approach to complementary techniques is vital if they are to be integrated into practice.

References

Adams AK (1996). Use of placebo in studies of postoperative vomiting is unethical. *British Medical Journal* **313**, 233.

Allen DL, Kitching AJ & Nagle C (1994). P6 acupressure and nausea and vomiting after gynaecological surgery. *Anaesthesia and Intensive Care* **22**, 691–3.

Al-Sadi M, Newman B & Julious SA (1997). Acupuncture in the prevention of postoperative nausea and vomiting. *Anaesthesia* **52**, 658–61.

Anon (1995). Risking the alternatives. *Health Which*, pp.196–9.

Arfen Z, Owen H, Plummer J L *et al.* (1995). A double blind randomised trial of ginger for the prevention of postoperative nausea and vomiting. *Anaesthesia and Intensive Care* **23**, 449–52.

Barsoum G, Perry EP & Fraser IA (1990). Postoperative vomiting is relieved by acupressure. *Journal of the Royal Society of Medicine* **83**, 86–9.

Bone ME, Wilkinson DJ, Young JR *et al.* (1990). Ginger root – a new antiemetic. The effect of ginger root on postoperative nausea and vomiting after major gynaecological surgery. *Anaesthesia* **45**, 669–71.

Dundee JW & Ghaly RG (1989). Does the timing of P6 acupuncture influence its efficacy as a postoperative antiemetic? *British Journal of Anaesthesia* **63**, 630P.

Dundee JW & Ghaly RG (1991). Local anaesthesia blocks the antiemetic action of P6. *Clinical Pharmacology and Therapeutics* **50**, 78–80.

Dundee J W & Young J (1990). Prophylactic antiemetic action of acupuncture in patients having cancer chemotherapy. *Journal of the Royal Society of Medicine* **83**, 360–2.

Dundee JW, Chestnutt WN, Ghaly RG *et al.* (1986). Traditional Chinese acupuncture: a potentially useful antiemetic? *British Medical Journal* **293**, 583–4.

Eberhart L H, Doring H J, Holzrichter P *et al.* (1998). Therapeutic suggestions given during neuroleptanaesthesia decrease postoperative nausea and vomiting. *European Journal of Anaesthesiology* **15**, 446–52.

Elhakim M, el-Sebiae S, Kaschef N *et al.* (1998). Intravenous fluid and postoperative nausea and vomiting after daycase termination of pregnancy. *Acta Anaesthesiologica Scandinavica* **42**, 216–9.

Enqvist B, Bjorklund C, Engman M *et al.* (1997). Preoperative hypnosis reduces postoperative vomiting after surgery of the breasts. *Acta Anaesthesiologica Scandinavica* **41**, 1028–32.

Evans C & Richardson PH (1988). Improved recovery and reduced postoperative stay after therapeutic suggestions during general anaesthesia. *Lancet* **2**, 491–3.

Fan CF, Tanhiu E, Joshi S *et al.* (1997). Acupressure treatment for prevention of postoperative nausea and vomiting. *Anesthesia and Analgesia* **84**, 821–5.

Fassoulaki A, Papils K, Sarantopoulos C *et al.* (1993). Transcutaneous electrical nerve stimulation reduces the incidence of vomiting after hysterectomy. *Anaesthesia and Analgesia* **76**, 1012–14.

Faymonville ME, Fissette J, Mambourg PH *et al.* (1995). Hypnosis as an adjunct therapy in conscious sedation for plastic surgery. *Regional Anaesthesia* **20**, 145–51.

Fischer-Rasmussen W, Kjaer SK, Dahl C *et al.* (1991). Ginger treatment of hyperemesis gravidarum. *European Journal of Obstetrics, Gynaecology and Reproductive Biology* **38**, 19–24.

Fry ENS (1986). Acupressure and postoperative vomiting. *Anaesthesia* **41**, 661–2.

Gieron C, Wieland B, von der Laage D *et al.* (1993). Acupressure in the prevention of postoperative nausea and vomiting. *Anaesthetist* **42**, 221–6.

Goodwin AP, Rowe WL, Ogg TW *et al.* (1991). Oral fluids prior to day surgery. The effect of shortening the preoperative fluid fast on postoperative morbidity. *Anaesthesia* **46**, 1066–8.

Ho CM, Hseu SS, Tsai SK *et al.* (1996). Effect of P6 acupressure on prevention of nausea and vomiting after epidural morphine for post-Cesarean section pain relief. *Acta Anaesthesiologica Scandinavica* **40**, 372–5.

Hovorjka J, Korttilla K & Erkola O (1990). The experience of the person ventilating the lungs does influence postoperative nausea and vomiting. *Acta Anaesthesiologica Scandinavica* **34**, 2035.

Hovorjka J, Korttila K & Erkola O (1990). Gastric aspiration at the end of anaesthesia does not decrease postoperative nausea and vomiting. *Anaesthesia and Intensive Care* **18**, 58–61.

Kaptchuk T J, Edwards RA & Eisenberg D M (1996). Complementary medicine: efficacy beyond the placebo effect. In *Complementary medicine: an objective appraisal* (ed. E Ernst), pp.42–70. Butterworth Heinemann, Oxford.

Kearney R, Mack C & Entwhistle L (1998). Withholding oral fluids from children undergoing day surgery reduces vomiting. *Paediatric Anaesthesia* **8**, 331–6.

Lauder GR, McQuillan PJ & Pickering RM (1995). Psychological adjuncts to postoperative anti-emesis. *British Journal of Anaesthesia* **74**, 266–70.

Lewis IH, Pryn SJ, Reynolds PI *et al.* (1991). Effect of P6 acupressure on postoperative vomiting in children undergoing outpatient strabismus correction. *British Journal of Anaesthesia* **67**, 73–8.

Lui WH, Standen PJ & Aitkenhead AR (1992). Therapeutic suggestions during general anaesthesia in patients undergoing hysterectomy. *British Journal of Anaesthesia* **68**, 277–81.

McMillan CM (1994). Transcutaneous electrical stimulation of Neiguan antiemetic acupuncture point in controlling sickness following opioid analgesia in major orthopaedic surgery. *Physiotherapy* **80**, 59.

Maroof M, Ahmed SM, Khan RM *et al.* (1997). Intraoperative suggestions reduce incidence of posthysterectomy emesis. *Journal of Pakistani Medical Association* **47**, 202–4.

Oddby-Muhrbeck E, Jakobsson J & Enqvist B (1995). Implicit processing and therapeutic suggestion during balanced anaesthesia. *Acta Anaesthesiologica Scandinavica* **39**, 333–7.

Phillips S, Ruggier R & Hutchinson SE (1993). *Zingiber officinale* (ginger) – an antiemetic for day case surgery. *Anaesthesia* **48**, 7157.

Rowbotham D J (1992). Current Management of postoperative nausea and vomiting. *British Journal of Anaesthesia* **69**(Suppl.1), 46S–59S.

Saks M (1991). The flight from science? The reporting of acupuncture in British mainstream journals from 1800 to 1990. *Complementary Medicine Research* **5**, 178–83.

Schlager A, Offer T & Baldissera I (1998). Laser stimulation of acupuncture point P6 reduces postoperative vomiting in children undergoing strabismus surgery. *British Journal of Anaesthesia* **81**, 529–33.

Schwager KL, Baines DB & Meyer RJ (1996). Acupuncture and postoperative vomiting in day-stay paediatric patients. *Anaesthesia and Intensive Care* **24**, 674–7.

Sharma SS & Gupta YK (1998). Reversal of cisplatin-induced delay in gastric emptying in rats by ginger. *Journal of Ethnopharmacology* **62**, 49–55.

Stein DJ, Birnbach DJ, Danzer BI *et al.* (1997). Acupressure versus intravenous metoclopramide to prevent nausea and vomiting during spinal anaesthesia for cesarean section. *Anesthesia and Analgesia* **84**, 342–5.

Tate S (1997). Peppermint oil: a treatment for postoperative nausea. *Journal of Advanced Nursing* **26**, 543–9.

ter Reit G, Kleijnen J & Knipschild P (1990). Acupuncture and chronic pain: a criterion based meta-analysis. *Journal of Clinical Epidemiology* **43**, 1191–9.

Trepanier CA & Isabel L (1993). Perioperative gastric aspiration increases postoperative nausea and vomiting in outpatients. *Canadian Journal of Anaesthesia* **40**, 325–6.

Vickers AJ (1996). Can acupuncture have specific effects on health? A systematic review of acupuncture antiemesis trials. *Journal of the Royal Society of Medicine* **89**, 303–11.

Visalyaputra S, Petchpaisit N, Somcharoen K *et al.* (1998). The efficacy of ginger root in the prevention of postoperative nausea and vomiting after outpatient gynaecological laparoscopy. *Anaesthesia* **53**, 506–10.

Williams AR, Hind M, Sweeney BP *et al.* (1994). The incidence and severity of postoperative nausea and vomiting in patients exposed to positive intra-operative suggestions. *Anaesthesia* **49**, 340–2.

Chapter 5

What if anti-emetic therapy fails?

David J Rowbotham

Introduction

PONV is regarded by many patients as the most unpleasant potential side-effect after surgery and anaesthesia. Many anaesthetists are aware of this and will routinely administer or prescribe an anti-emetic drug routinely. Despite this practice, many patients will experience troublesome PONV. In this chapter, we will explore factors influencing failure of initial treatment and consider further therapeutic options. The use of combination therapy will be reviewed also.

There are two situations when failure of treatment becomes apparent. First, in an individual patient complaining of PONV despite anti-emetic therapy. Second, a high incidence of PONV may become apparent in a population of patients, perhaps after clinical audit. Although many similar factors apply to both situations, we will consider them separately.

Failure of treatment in an individual patient

There are various factors to be aware of when treatment in an individual patient has failed.

Has the drug been given?

In many cases, this may be the most important single factor in failure of treatment when an anti-emetic has been prescribed for post-operative use. There is evidence that anti-emetic therapy has a relatively low priority on the ward and that the utilisation of anti-emetic drugs by medical and nursing staff could be improved. This problem is discussed in detail in Chapter 8.

Has the drug been absorbed?

In most cases, anti-emetics are given intravenously or intramuscularly but they may be given orally, perhaps as pre-medication or on discharge after day-case surgery. In this situation, oral bioavailability and rate of absorption may be an important factor in the failure of treatment.

Table 5.1 summarises the bioavailability and time to maximum plasma concentration (t_{max}) of some anti-emetics after oral administration. Data in the literature are often limited, particularly for the older anti-emetics (Rowbotham 1992). Metoclopramide is absorbed rapidly and the mean (range) t_{max} in volunteers is 0.9 (0.5–1.25) h (Ross-Lee *et al.* 1981). However, despite a bioavailability of 80 per cent, there is an enormous individual variation. For example, some subjects absorb only one third of the oral dose (Harrington *et al.* 1983). Prochlorperazine is poorly absorbed (t_{max} range 1.5–5 h (Taylor *et al.* 1987), bioavailability 15 per cent (Isah *et al.* 1992)). Data with respect to cyclizine are sparse. In one volunteer, t_{max} of 2 h was observed after administration of oral cyclizine 50 mg (Roila & Delfavero 1995). Ondansetron is quite well absorbed orally with a bioavailability of about 60 per cent and a t_{max} of 0.5–2 h (Roila & Delfavero 1995). Dolasetron is rapidly converted to its major metabolite (hydrodolasetron) which is active at the 5-HT_3 receptor (Blafour & Goa 1997). Median t_{max} of the metabolite after oral administration was approximately 1 h (Boxenbaum *et al.* 1993).

These data are from patients or volunteers with normal gastric emptying. In the peri-operative period, many factors delay, or even inhibit completely, gastric emptying (Table 5.2). Opioid administration is particularly important in this context. Clearly, in the peri-operative period, the absorption of any anti-emetic administered orally may be unreliable.

Has the appropriate dose been administered?

The drug may be ineffective because an inappropriate dose has been administered. With the exception of droperidol, only the recently introduced anti-emetic drugs have undergone extensive dose–response investigation. The recommended doses of cyclizine, prochlorperazine and metoclopramide have not been derived from appropriate dose-ranging studies, primarily because they were introduced before strict licensing regulations. However, evidence suggests that metoclopramide is relatively ineffective because the recommended dose (10 mg) is insufficient (Rowbotham 1992; Henzi *et al.* 1999). The dose–response relationship of droperidol has been investigated in a number of clinical situations in an attempt to separate the anti-emetic effect from sedation (Rowbotham 1992).

Drugs introduced more recently, such as ondansetron and dolasetron, have undergone extensive investigation before licensing. Recommended doses are derived from specifically designed dose-ranging studies. However, even these data are often not clear-cut. For example, data from original studies on ondansetron suggested that a dose of 8 mg (rather than that of the recommended 4 mg) may be more appropriate for those with a previous history of PONV (McKenzie *et al.* 1993).

Table 5.1 Oral absorption of some anti-emetics

	Bioavailability (%)	t_{max} *(h)*	*Reference*
Metoclopramide	80 Range (32–97)	1–2.5	Ross-Lee *et al.* 1981; Harrington *et al.* 1983
Prochlorperazine	15	2.8	Taylor & Bateman 1987
Cyclizine		2	Griffin & Baselt 1984
Ondansetron	60	0.5–2	Roila & Delfavero 1995
Dolasetron		1*	Boxenbaum *et al.* 1993
Granisetron		1.5–1.9	Kudoh *et al.* 1993

*active metabolite

Table 5.2 Important causes of delayed gastric emptying in the peri-operative period

Physiological
- Pain
- Anxiety

Pathological
- GI tract obstruction
- Acute gastritis
- Electrolyte imbalance
- Diabetes

Pharmacological
- Opioids
  - μ agonists
  - partial agonists
  - mixed agonist/antagonists
- Anticholinergics
- Sympathomimetics

Is the drug still present?

The elimination half-lives of the commonly used anti-emetics vary widely (Table 5.3) and data are again sparse with respect to the older drugs. Metoclopramide has a half-life of approximately 4 h (Harrington *et al.* 1983). The pharmacokinetics of prochlorperazine were published years after its introduction into clinical practice (Taylor & Bateman 1987; Isah *et al.* 1992; Nahata *et al.* 1992). Its half-life is longer than that of metoclopramide, although a study in children receiving chemotherapy revealed a large range (1.2–15.5 h). The limited data available indicate that cyclizine has a comparatively long half-life (Griffin & Baselt 1984; Walker & Kanfer 1996) compared with other anti-emetics. The elimination half-life of droperidol is approximately 2 h (Cressman *et al.* 1973; Grumwald *et al.* 1993).

Table 5.3 Half-lives of some anti-emetics

	Half-life (h)	*Reference*
Metoclopramide	4	Harrington *et al.* (1983)
Prochlorperazine	6.8	Taylor & Bateman (1987)
	7.5	Isah *et al.* (1992)
	5.6 *	Nahata *et al.* (1992)
	Range 1.2–15.5*	
Droperidol	2	Cressman *et al.* (1973); Fischler *et al.* (1986)
	1.7 *	Cressman *et al.* 1973
Cyclizine	13	Walker & Kanfer (1996)
	24**	Griffin & Baselt (1984)
Ondansetron	3.8	Roila & Delfavero (1995)
Dolasetron (active metabolite)	6.6–8.8	Dimmitt *et al.* (1999)
Granisetron	2.9–6.3	Kudoh *et al.* (1993); Allen *et al.* (1994)

* children
** in 1 volunteer only

The pharmacokinetics of the new 5-HT_3 antagonists are well described. For example, the elimination half-life of ondansetron is approximately 4 h (Roila & Delfavero 1995) and that of the active metabolite of dolasetron is 6.6-8.8 h (Dimmitt *et al.* 1999).

Despite the fact that anti-emetics are often ineffective, our knowledge of the pharmacokinetics of many anti-emetics is superficial. For example, there are few data available on the pharmacokinetics of infusion regimens and the time course of effector-site concentrations. More work is required in this area.

Is there a treatable cause for PONV?

One of the most important principles of medical practice is to treat the cause of a symptom before treating the symptom itself. There are many causes of PONV and several are treatable and potentially serious. It may be that the anti-emetic therapy has failed because a potent cause of PONV is present – all patients who do not respond to anti-emetic therapy should be assessed with this in mind.

Table 5.4 summarises the causes of PONV. Hypotension and hypoxaemia are common and important complications after anaesthesia and surgery. A frequent cause of PONV, particularly in the day-care setting, is optimistic fluid intake or mobilisation. If these are included as criteria for discharge, it may be that they are introduced at an inappropriately early stage in the patient's recovery. Psychological factors play an important role also and, if predominant, will often be associated with poor response to therapy. Occasionally, failure to respond to treatment may indicate abdominal or other pathology resulting from a surgical complication. This should be considered in all poor- or non-responders, particularly before discharge from the day-care unit.

Table 5.4 Important causes of PONV

Hypotension	
Hypoxaemia	
Drugs	– opioids
	– antibiotics
GI pathology	
Psychological factors	
Mobilisation	
Fluid intake	
Nasogastric tube	
Pain	

Opioids are a common cause of PONV, especially if these drugs are being administered injudiciously. A more appropriate post-operative pain regimen may reduce the problem significantly. It should be remembered that other drugs can cause nausea and vomiting and, in the peri-operative period, antibiotics are a common culprit. The use of these drugs should be reassessed if PONV is a severe problem.

What drug to use next?

Despite the factors discussed above, the great majority of patients in whom an anti-emetic has failed will require the administration of another anti-emetic. It is probably appropriate to choose a drug which acts by a different mechanism. This statement is not based on evidence from clinical trials in this situation because these data do not exist. However, there are some data regarding combination of anti-emetics for PONV prophylaxis (see below) and the strategy is consistent with the basic, well-accepted, pharmacological principles.

Table 5.5 summarises the sites of action of anti-emetics and the pharmacology of many of these drugs is discussed in Chapter 3. Metoclopramide, droperidol and prochlorperazine act primarily at the dopamine receptor and all are associated with extrapyramidal side-effects. Cyclizine is predominantly anticholinergic. The 5-HT_3 antagonists, such as ondansetron, dolasetron and granisetron, are relatively effective and well tolerated and represent another group of drugs with a specific site of action. Antagonists at the NK_1 receptor are also anti-emetics and may be a useful therapeutic alternative in future (Minami *et al.* 1998; Fukuda *et al.* 1999). Presently, these drugs are not licensed but are undergoing clinical trials for PONV.

Dexamethasone has been shown to be an effective anti-emetic for the prophylaxis of PONV (Lopez-Olaondo *et al.* 1996). It is not used widely as yet, but it may be useful when initial anti-emetic therapy has failed. It has been used successfully in combination with other anti-emetics (see below). The use of cannabinoids for nausea and vomiting associated with chemotherapy is well established (Dalzell *et al.* 1986) but there are no consistent data confirming efficacy for PONV (Lewis *et al.* 1994).

Table 5.5 Sites of action of anti-emetics

Antagonists
Dopaminergic
Cholinergic
Histaminergic
$5\text{-}HT_3$
NK_1
Agonists
Steroids
Cannabinoids

In theory, they may offer an alternative when initial therapy has failed but the clinician has available several other well-established options.

Non-pharmacological methods

Acupuncture has been shown to be effective for the treatment of PONV and is reviewed in some detail in Chapter 4. Vickers (1996) analysed 33 studies investigating acupuncture administered during general anaesthesia (n=4) or when awake (n=29). Clinical situations included PONV (n=21), morning sickness (n=7) and chemotherapy (n=5). In those studies where acupuncture was administered to the awake patient (n=29), 27 showed acupuncture to be effective. Therefore, the literature suggests that acupuncture may be a useful therapeutic tool when initial therapy has failed.

Failure of anti-emetic prophylaxis in a patient population

Clinical audit or simple clinical impression may indicate that the incidence of PONV in a certain population of patients is unacceptably high despite the administration of an anti-emetic drug. We now discuss the options available in this situation.

Organisational factors

This is a very common cause for the failure of anti-emetic prophylaxis in a group of patients, as well as in any individual patient (see above). This is discussed in detail in Chapter 8.

Choice of drug and dose

There is a wealth of literature concerning the efficacy of anti-emetics in the prophylaxis of PONV in many types of surgery. However, it is not possible to make conclusions regarding the relative efficacy of these drugs with respect to type of surgery. It would make sense to change the drug if the first-choice medication was ineffective and this should be done taking into account the principles discussed above. The question of dose has been considered.

Combination therapy

If there are no organisational problems and it is thought that an appropriate drug in a suitable dose has proven ineffective, then combination therapy should be considered. Presently, there is considerable interest in this in the literature. However, many data have been published in abstract form and some studies do not allow direct comparison of each individual drug with the combination. In these studies, the combination group is not compared directly with groups receiving each of the two drugs used in combination. Many compare the combination with one other group only. In general, most have found combinations more efficacious than a single drug.

Some of the studies investigating a combination of ondansetron and droperidol are summarised in Table 5.6. One of the first was by Pueyo *et al.* (1996) who studied females undergoing intra-abdominal surgery (75 per cent gynaecological). Anti-emetic therapy was given in a randomised double-blind manner at, and 12 h after, induction of anaesthesia. There were four groups: placebo then placebo; droperidol 2.5 mg then droperidol 1.25 mg; ondansetron 4 mg then placebo; droperidol 2.5 mg plus ondansetron 4 mg then droperidol 1.25 mg. Ondansetron and droperidol were superior to placebo but the combination was significantly more effective than monotherapy. For example, at 12 h, the incidence of nausea was 8 per cent in the combination group compared with 28 and 40 per cent in the droperidol and ondansetron groups, respectively. A similar pattern was observed up to 48 h post-operatively. The overall incidence of PONV remained 8 per cent in the combination group compared with 40 and 44 per cent in the droperidol and ondansetron groups, respectively.

The comparative efficacy of combinations of droperidol and ondansetron has been compared when given as a mixture within a patient-controlled analgesia (PCA) syringe. Wrench *et al.* (1996) investigated 60 patients undergoing gynaecological surgery and post-operative PCA (morphine 1 mg/ml). Patients were randomised to receive three anti-emetic regimens: (i) ondansetron 4 mg bolus plus ondansetron 8 mg per 60-ml syringe; (ii) droperidol 1.25 mg plus droperidol 3 mg per 60 ml-syringe; and (iii) a combination of both drugs as a bolus plus both drugs added to the syringe. There was a relatively low incidence of PONV in all groups in this study but, at 12 h post-operatively, the incidence of nausea in the combination group was 5 per cent compared with 20 and 25 per cent in the droperidol and ondansetron groups, respectively ($p<0.05$).

Several studies have shown not only efficacy of dexamethasone for the prevention of PONV but also increased efficacy when used in combination with ondansetron (Table 5.7). For example, Splinter & Rhine (1998) gave children undergoing squint surgery one of two anti-emetic regimens in a randomised double-blind manner: ondansetron 150 μg/kg (maximum 8 mg) or ondansetron 50 μg/kg plus dexamethasone 150 μg/kg (maximum 8 mg). The design of this study was not ideal, as discussed above, but the incidence of vomiting at 24 h was 28 per cent in the ondansetron group compared with 9 per cent in the combination group. Furthermore, no children in the combination group vomited on the way home.

Table 5.6 Droperidol/ondansetron combinations

Reference	*Combinations*	*Surgery*	*Results*
Pueyo *et al.* (1996)	Ondan Drop Drop + ondan	Major gynae PCA	Improved
Wrench *et al.* (1996)	Ondan Drop Drop + ondan	Major gynae PCA	Improved (first 12 h only)
Riley *et al.* (1998)	Drop Drop + ondan	Major gynae	Improved
Klockgether Radke *et al.* (1997)	Drop Ondan Drop + ondan	Paediatric strabismus	No improvement

Table 5.7 Ondansetron/dexamethasone combinations

Reference	*Combinations*	*Surgery*	*Results*
McKenzie *et al.* (1994)	Ondan Ondan + dexameth	Major gynae	Improved
Lopez-Olaondo *et al.* (1996)	Ondan Dexamethasone Ondan + dexameth	Major gynae	Improved
Splinter & Rhine (1998)	Ondan Ondan + dexameth	Paediatric strabismus	Improved

Ondan = ondansetron
Drop = droperidol
PCA = patient-controlled analgesia
Dexameth = dexamethasone

Lopez-Olaondo *et al.* (1996) investigated patients undergoing major gynaecological surgery in a study of good design. Anti-emetics were given at induction of anaesthesia: placebo, ondansetron 4 mg, dexamethasone 8 mg, or a combination of dexamethasone 8 mg and ondansetron 4 mg. Both ondansetron and dexamethasone were significantly better than placebo but the combination was significantly more efficacious than all groups. For example, the incidence of nausea at 24 h was 48 per cent in the ondansetron group and 40 per cent in the dexamethasone group compared with 76 per cent in the placebo group. The incidence of nausea in the combination group was only 12 per cent.

As yet, there are insufficient data from studies of good design published in full to arrive at a comprehensive picture with regard to combination therapy. However, initial data are promising and considerable work is ongoing at present.

The future of anti-emetic therapy

There is considerable potential for improving our success in preventing and treating PONV. Perhaps, with the introduction of new drugs, the problem of the patient who has not responded to anti-emetic therapy will be infrequent. We live in hope. Perhaps an appropriate way forward is to improve the use of presently available anti-emetics. There is plenty of scope for this and advances can be made by any clinician with an interest in this area. Finally, there is a parallel with the accepted concept of balanced analgesia. It is likely that efficacy can be improved with the use of several anti-emetics, each acting at a different site.

References

Allen A, Asgill CC, Pierce DM, Upward J & Zussman BD (1994). Pharmacokinetics and tolerability of ascending intravenous doses of granisetron, a novel 5-HT3 antagonist, in healthy human subjects. *European Journal of Clinical Pharmacology* **46**, 159–62.

Balfour JA & Goa KL (1997). Dolasetron – A review of its pharmacology and therapeutic potential in the management of nausea and vomiting induced by chemotherapy, radiotherapy or surgery. *Drugs* **54**, 273–98.

Boxenbaum H, Gillespie T, Heck K & Hahne W (1993). Human dolasetron pharmacokinetics. 2. Absorption and disposition following single-dose oral-administration to normal-male subjects. *Biopharmaceutics & Drug Disposition* **14**, 131–41.

Cressman WA, Plostnieks J & Johnson PC (1973). Absorption, metabolism and excretion of droperidol by human subjects following intramuscular and intravenous administration. *Anesthesiology* **38**, 363–9.

Dalzell AM, Bartlett H & Lilleyman JS (1986). Nabilone: an alternative antiemetic for cancer chemotherapy. *Archives of Disease in Childhood* **61**, 502–5.

Dimmitt DC, Choo YS, Martin LA, Arumugham T, Hahne WF & Weir SJ (1999). Intravenous pharmacokinetics and absolute oral bioavailability of dolasetron in healthy volunteers: Part 1. *Biopharmaceutics & Drug Disposition* **20**, 29–39.

Fischler M, Bonnet F, Trang H *et al.* (1986). The pharmacokinetics of droperidol in anesthetized patients. *Anesthesiology* **64**, 486–9.

Fukuda H, Koga T, Furukawa N, Nakamura E & Shiroshita Y (1999). The tachykinin NK1 receptor antagonist GR205171 abolishes the retching activity of neurons comprising the central pattern generator for vomiting in dogs. *Neuroscience Research* **33**, 25–32.

Griffin DS & Baselt RC (1984). Blood and urine concentrations of cyclizine by nitrogen-phosphorus gas-liquid chromatography. *Journal of Analytical Toxicology* **8**, 97–9.

Grunwald Z, Torjman M, Schieren H & Bartkowski RR (1993). The pharmacokinetics of droperidol in anesthetized children. *Anesthesia and Analgesia* **76**,1238–42.

Harrington RA, Hamilton CW, Brogden RN, Linkewich JA, Romankiewicz JA & Heel RC (1983). Metoclopramide: An updated review of its pharmacological properties and clinical use. *Drugs* **25**, 451–94.

Henzi I, Walder B & Tramer MR (1999). Metoclopramide in the prevention of postoperative nausea and vomiting: A quantitative systematic review of randomised placebo controlled trials. *British Journal of Anaesthesia* (in press).

Isah AO, Rawlins MD & Bateman DN (1992). The pharmacokinetics and effects of prochlorperazine in elderly female volunteers. *Age and Ageing* **21**, 27–31.

KlockgetherRadke A, Neumann S, Neumann P, Braun U & Muhlendyck H (1997). Ondansetron, droperidol and their combination for the prevention of post-operative vomiting in children. *European Journal of Anaesthesiology* **14**, 362–7.

Kudoh S, Okada H, Miyazaki R *et al.* (1993). A phase I study of granisetron hydrochloride (2) – Pharmacokinetics of granisetron following single oral administration in healthy Japanese subjects. *Japanese Pharmacology & Therapeutics* **21**, 169–76.

Lewis IH, Campbell DN & Barrowcliffe MP (1994). Effect of nabilone on nausea and vomiting after total abdominal hysterectomy. *British Journal of Anaesthesia* **73**, 244–6.

Lopez-Olaondo L, Carrascosa F, Pueyo FJ, Monedero P, Busto N & Saez A (1996). Combination of ondansetron and dexamethasone in the prophylaxis of postoperative nausea and vomiting. *British Journal of Anaesthesia* **76**, 835–40.

McKenzie R, Kovac A, O'Connor T *et al.* (1993). Comparison of ondansetron versus placebo to prevent postoperative nausea and vomiting in women undergoing ambulatory gynecologic surgery. *Anesthesiology* **78**, 21–8.

McKenzie R, Tantisira B, Karambelkar DJ, Riley TJ & Abdelhady H (1994). Comparison of ondansetron with ondansetron plus dexamethasone in the prevention of postoperative nausea and vomiting. *Anesthesia & Analgesia* **79**, 961–4.

Minami M, Endo T, Kikuchi K *et al.* (1998). Antiemetic effects of sendide, a peptide tachykinin NK1 receptor antagonist, in the ferret. *European Journal of Pharmacology* **363**, 49–55.

Nahata MC, Ford C & Ruymann FB (1992). Pharmacokinetics and safety of prochlorperazine in pediatric patients receiving cancer chemotherapy. *Journal of Clinical Pharmacy and Therapeutics* **17**, 121–3.

Pueyo FJ, Carrascosa F, Lopez L, Iribarren MJ, Garcia Pedrajas F & Saez A (1996). Combination of ondansetron and droperidol in the prophylaxis of postoperative nausea and vomiting. *Anesthesia and Analgesia* **83**, 117–22.

Riley TJ, McKenzie R, Tantisira BR & Hamilton DL (1998). Droperidol-ondansetron combination versus droperidol alone for postoperative control of emesis after total abdominal hysterectomy. *Journal of Clinical Anesthesia* **10**, 6–12.

Roila F & Delfavero A (1995). Ondansetron clinical pharmacokinetics. *Clinical Pharmacokinetics* **29**, 95–109.

Ross-Lee LM, Hooper WD & Bochner F (1981). Single-dose pharmacokinetics of metoclopramide. *European Journal of Pharmacology* **20**, 465–71.

Rowbotham DJ (1992). Current management of postoperative nausea and vomiting. *British Journal of Anaesthesia* **69**, 46S–59S.

Splinter WM & Rhine EJ (1998). Low-dose ondansetron with dexamethasone more effectively decreases vomiting after strabismus surgery in children than does high-dose ondansetron. *Anesthesiology* **88**, 72–5.

Taylor WB & Bateman DN (1987). Preliminary studies of the pharmacokinetics and pharmacodynamics of prochlorperazine in healthy volunteers. *British Journal of Clinical Pharmacology* **23**, 137–42.

Vickers AJ (1996). Can acupunture have specific effects on health? A systematic review of acupuncture antiemetic trials. *Journal of the Royal Society of Medicine* **89**, 303–11.

Walker RB & Kanfer I (1996). Pharmacokinetics of cyclizine following intravenous administration to human volunteers. *European Journal of Pharmaceutical Sciences* **4**, 301–6.

Wrench LJ, Ward JH, Walder AD & Hobbs GJ (1996). The prevention of postoperative nausea and vomiting using a combination of ondansetron and droperidol. *Anaesthesia* **51**, 776–8.

Chapter 6

Pharmaceutical considerations in the preparation and administration of anti-emetic agents

Philip Howard

Introduction

About 56 per cent (Anon 1993) of the four million patients that have operations in UK hospitals every year (Anon 1998) are given anti-emetics to treat or prevent PONV. Of these, most are prescribed as intramuscular, 'p.r.n.' injections on ward areas or are given intravenous boluses or infusions within the operating-theatre complex. Anaesthetists will predominantly use the intravenous route and nurses the intramuscular route. This procedure is so routine that probably very little thought goes into the process. However, a large number of issues are involved in this process, and these will be discussed in this chapter.

The main elements of the process and their related issues can be divided as follows:

- *Preparation of anti-emetics*
  - particulate contamination and its prevention
  - microbiological contamination and its prevention
  - labelling of syringes
  - compatibility of admixtures
  - stability of infusions.

- *Administration of anti-emetics*
  - route and adverse effects
  - rate of injection.

Preparation of anti-emetics

Particulate contamination in intravenous medication

All injectable medication contains particulate contamination; this can be classified into intrinsic and extrinsic contamination, depending on its origin (see Table 6.1).

Table 6.1 Sources of particulate contamination

Intrinsic	*Extrinsic*
Metal	Rubber
Glass	Plastic
Cotton	Glass
Barium sulphate	Cotton
	Precipitates

Intrinsic contamination

Intrinsic contamination arises during the manufacturing process, transport and storage. In 1973, the British Pharmacopoeia (BP) introduced limits for the particulate matter allowed in large-volume fluids. These limits were not based on any clinical evidence of the harmful effects of infused particles. Filtration during the manufacturing process allowed these limits to be easily met. However, the BP did not set limits for particulate matter for small volume fluids (less than 100 ml) or freeze-dried powders. The United States Pharmacopoeia (USP) set limits for both large- and small-volume fluids (see Table 6.2).

Studies into the intrinsic particulate contamination of small-volume fluids showed that there is large variation in total particle counts between different drugs, but also between different batches of the same drug (Backhouse *et al.* 1987). More astonishingly, the particulate matter in freeze-dried drugs after reconstitution in a carrier fluid was found to be up to ten times more than those drugs already in solution.

Intrinsic contamination can also be generated by interaction between the drug and its container during transportation and storage.

Extrinsic contamination

Extrinsic contamination is generated through the various manipulations involved in administering drugs and infusions. When an ampoule is opened, glass particles are released. Many of these are visible, i.e. >40 μm, but many others are not. The glass particles fall back into the ampoule and are drawn up through the needle into the syringe (Shaw & Lyall 1985) A 0.2 μm end-line filter has been shown to eliminate these particles (Sabon *et al.* 1989). Cores of rubber bungs can be released when a needle pierces a bung. Particles of plastic are also released from administration equipment, such as giving sets and syringes (Taylor 1982). The introduction by some pharmaceutical companies of the plastic (polypropylene) flexi-amp is progress towards fewer particles, especially when the use of filters outside of intensive care areas is minimal in many hospitals.

If drugs are physically incompatible, they may precipitate out into solution generating many more particles.

Table 6.2 Particulate matter standards

British & European Pharmacopoeias		
Large-volume parenterals (>100 ml)		
No more than	1000/ml	>2 µm
No more than	100/ml	>5 µm
United States Pharmacopoeia		
Large-volume parenterals (>100 ml)		
No more than	50/ml	<10 µm
No more than	5/ml	<5 µm
Small-volume parenterals (<100 ml)		
No more than	1,000 per container	<25 µm
No visible particles should be present		

Table 6.3 Size of particulate matter

	µm
Blood set filter	200
Human hair	120
Visual limits	80
Industry standard filter	15
Blood corpuscle	7.5
Small blood capillary	5
Chylomicron	4
Candida (yeast)	2
Spores	1.2+
Bacteria	0.2+
Virus	0.1

Clinical consequences of particulate infusion

The clinical effects of particulate matter can be divided into two parts: local effects and systemic effects. Local effects involve irritation of the vein at the cannula entry site (phlebitis). Systemic effects result from the particles being removed from the circulation by various organs, especially the lungs.

Phlebitis

Phlebitis is a common adverse effect of intravenous therapy and the effects can last for many weeks after therapy. Up to 50 per cent of patients get phlebitis (Falchuk *et al.* 1985). Patient groups where intravenous access is difficult can have a lot of discomfort from regular cannulae changes that are short-lived because of phlebitis.

Many factors have been implicated in infusion phlebitis. Infection is often thought to be the main cause, but is rare with less than 1 per cent of catheter tips being successfully cultured (Francombe 1998). It appears that particulate contamination is the major culprit, but the use of microfilters can reduce the incidence of phlebitis by 50 per cent (Allcutt *et al.* 1983). Table 6.4 shows common causes of infusion-related phlebitis.

Systemic effects

Particles with a diameter of 7–12 μm that are injected into the systemic circulation are usually removed by the pulmonary capillary bed. Larger particles become trapped and undergo phagocytosis, if biodegradable; if not, a granuloma is formed, surrounded by mononucleocytes and foreign body giant cells with a fibrous sheath around the outside. The use of end-line filters has shown a lower ESR and WCC (De Luca *et al.* 1976).

Accidental air emboli

These can form in many different ways. Intravenous fluid on warming up from cool storage can release small bubbles. Also, additional bubbles can arise from priming. Infusion of non-collapsible containers or accidental disconnection can also result in air entering the circulation. Fatalities can occur dependent upon the volume of air administered or the rate of infusion (Marshall & Lloyd 1987). The use of infusion pumps and 0.2 μm air venting filters can prevent this adverse effect.

Microbiogical contamination

This also can be separated into intrinsic and extrinsic contamination. Intrinsic contamination is microbiological contamination during the manufacturing and transport process. This is very rare. Guidelines are in place for intravenous fluids and the giving sets that they flow to be changed every 24 hours, where possible, to prevent repetition of hospital-acquired sepsis related to contaminated intravenous fluids (Macmillan 1972).

Table 6.4 Possible causes of infusion-related phlebitis cannula type

Infusion pH
Infusion tonicity
Location of IV site
Duration of infusion
Infection
Particulate matter

Table 6.5 *In vivo* effects of particulate contamination

Systemic effects	*Local effects*
Inflammation	Phlebitis
Granulomata	
Thrombi	
Lung lesions	
ARDS	
Multi-organ failure	

Extrinsic contamination is the result of manipulations of the intravenous administration systems while in use. The usual sources of infection are three-way taps, injection ports and connecting taps (Clayton *et al.* 1985). When a needle pierces an injection port, a warm meniscus of fluid is left behind. This is an ideal environment for bacterial growth. Any subsequent injections through the port will also inject any inoculate into the patient. The rate of in-use contamination of intravenous fluids ranges from 0 to 30 per cent with an average value of 3 per cent (Marshall & Lloyd 1987). It has also been shown that Gram-negative bacteria can grow to large numbers within 24 hours in simple intravenous infusions at room temperature (e.g. *Klebsiella sp.* 10^5/ml in 5 per cent glucose with 24 hours) (Maki *et al.* 1971). Total parenteral nutrition is probably the most ideal growth medium, and many hospitals insist on a dedicated IV line for total parenteral nutrition (Ng *et al.* 1989; Twum-Danso *et al.* 1989). It has been demonstrated that 0.2 μm filters are required, as 0.45 μm filters have been penetrated by certain bacteria (Holmes *et al.* 1980). Clinically significant nosocomial bacteraemia occurs less in a surgical intensive care unit (ICU) with the use of 0.2 μm filters (Quercia *et al.* 1986). End-line IV filters need to be changed every 24 hours as Gram-negative bacteria start to autolyse and release significant amounts of endotoxin. Endotoxin infusion results in pyrogenic, toxic and inflammatory reactions (Wardle 1986). There are some negatively charged filters that can trap the positively charged endotoxins for periods of up to 96 hours (Baumgartner *et al.* 1986).

Problems with filters

Filters are ideal for preventing particulate and microbiological contamination from reaching the systemic circulation, but they can have drawbacks. Most drugs can be filtered, so long as they are completely soluble. Agents that are not filterable are those drugs formulated as suspensions or emulsions or those which are not fully dissolved in their solvent. Of the agents used or considered anti-emetic, propofol is the only one. Propofol is a fat emulsion and should not be passed through a filter smaller than 5 μm. Also of importance is the fact that many blood constituents are too large to go through 0.2 μm filters. Red blood cells are 7.5 μm and platelets are 2–4 μm in diameter so standard 0.2 μm filters cannot be used when administering these.

The problem of drugs binding to filters (sorption) has been studied extensively (Trissell 1998). Most drugs delivered at high concentrations or fast-flow rates through administration sets will not bind significantly. Most end-line filters have a dead space so anti-emetics that need to reach the systemic circulation quickly will need a flush after administration.

Labelling of anti-emetics

It is recommended that anti-emetics be prepared immediately before use (Anon 1998). If anti-emetics are drawn up within the anaesthetic room in advance to give to a patient, they should be clearly labelled. Most injections are clear, colourless solutions which are difficult to distinguish, so can easily be mixed up without correct or any labelling. There have been many fatalities associated with not labelling syringes (Cousins & Upton 1998). The operating theatres seem to be the worst affected for unlabelled syringes, often with the anaesthetist and ODA preparing drugs and leaving them unlabelled on the anaesthetic room bench (Cousins & Upton 1998).

Compatibility of admixtures

With the poor outcomes using monotherapy for anti-emetics, the use of dual or more combinations will become more common. Also, there will be clinical situations when there is a need for anti-emetics to be added to solutions or mixed with other drugs – for example:

- to reduce the number of intramuscular injections a patient receives (e.g. combining an opioid with an anti-emetic);
- when incorporating an anti-emetic into a patient-controlled analgesic system (e.g. morphine and droperidol syringes);
- in ICUs when drugs and infusions come together on a three-way tap before entering the patient. If any of these infusions or drugs are incompatible, they may come out of solution to form a precipitate of solid particles which may be gelatinous, crystalline or granular in nature. The end-line filter will protect the patient but the filter will be occluded.

Drug stability and compatibility are crucial elements in drug delivery. There are a number of reasons for physical drug incompatibility, including:

- imbalance of drugs dissolved in complex co-solvents when added to other solutions;
- drugs that are weak acids or bases are formulated at high or low pH values to keep them in solution. If the pH changes markedly on adding to another solution, the drug may come out of solution;

- precipitation due to formation of salts that are relatively insoluble (e.g. calcium and phosphates);
- formation of insoluble complexes with large organic anions and actions (e.g. heparin and aminoglycosides).

Sorption phenomena can also be subclassified into two sorts:

- adsorption of a drug to the surface of a container (e.g. glass or plastics in bags, administration sets or filters). This is only important if a drug is given in low concentrations or small amounts as the amount adsorbed may be significant. At higher amounts or concentrations, saturation of binding sites occurs and is less significant;
- absorption into the matrix of plastic containers and administration sets, especially PVC, is another source of drug loss for lipid soluble drugs in solution. Polypropylene and polyethylene do not have the same problem as they contain no or little phthalate plasticisers.

Compatibility of drugs is often classified into four distinct areas:

- the drug in a solution for infusion;
- the drug added to another drug in a solution for infusion;
- the drug added to another drug in a syringe for infusion;
- drugs mixing at a Y site before entering a patient.

The appendix to this chapter, on pages 82–93, outlines some of the compatibility issues for parenteral anti-emetics in use in the UK. Only drugs commonly used in combination are included. More detailed information regarding drug compatibility is available from standard texts such as Trissell (1998).

General guidelines on admixtures

To minimise risk with the mixing of anti-emetics with other agents, it is better to publicise a small range of compatible agents in the ICUs, theatres and wards. This is already provided by some medical filter companies (e.g. Pall Medical Ltd).

The newer agents, such as ondansetron, seem to have a lot of compatibility work undertaken on them, which is useful.

Administration of anti-emetics

In the post-operative period, anti-emetics are usually given by two routes: intravenous or intramuscular. The intravenous route is the better of the two routes because of its bioavailability and speed of onset. The intramuscular route is problematic and should only be used in situations when nurses are not approved to give drugs by the intravenous route. Measures should be taken within hospitals to enable nurses to give anti-emetics into running fluids or directly into cannulae.

Intramuscular route

This route is complicated by the variable bioavailability of the drugs administered. It can often be slow, erratic or incomplete. The site of injection also affects the speed of absorption: fastest from the deltoid muscle and slowest from the gluteal muscles. Blood flow to the muscles is reduced in circulatory collapse or if cardiac output is low and can thus reduce absorption even more (Aronson 1995). Although it is common practice to swab the injection site before injection, it is probably unnecessary (Dann 1969).

Adverse effects do arise from intramuscular injections. The most common being skin reactions at the site of injection. Those agents whose pH differs markedly from the surrounding tissue, and which are or contain chemical irritants are the most troublesome. Incorrect administration technique is usually the main cause (Uchegbu & Florence 1996). A small number (0.4 per cent) of patients complain of persistent pain, erythema, a weal, induration, subcutaneous fat nodules, haematoma, bleeding, or abscess. These are more common in children (23 per cent). Pain in the muscle can also occur, and is partly related to the volume of the injection, which should generally be no more than 2 ml into the arm or thigh, but up to 5 ml into gluteus maximus (Hipwell *et al.* 1984). Local muscle damage is common. A rise in serum creatine kinase occurs and increases with the volume and concentration of the solution injected. It is not known whether the drug or diluent is the main cause. Patients who are anticoagulated or receiving thrombolysis should not receive intramuscular injections.

Of the anti-emetics that cause injection-site complications, prochlorperazine (0.1 per cent) seems to be the most common, and promethazine has been implicated. These were probably linked to the difference in pH (Greenblatt & Allen 1978).

Intravenous route

A number of different problems arise with the intravenous route, including:

- intravenous delivery devices, such as patient-controlled analgesia pumps that sometimes contain anti-emetics as well as opioids, can malfunction (Whipple *et al.* 1994);
- there may be particulate contamination (see above);
- there may be microbiological contamination (see above);
- problems with preservatives used in intravenous delivery systems – deaths have been reported in neonates and children from metabolic acidosis from benzoic alcohol preservatives (these are not used in any anti-emetics);
- solubilisers used in intravenous injections have caused anaphylactic reactions, other hypersensitivity reactions such as hyperventilation, hypoxia and pruritus,

and thrombophlebitis. Again these are not used in any anti-emetic agents. Propofol was formulated in cremaphor but is no longer. Pain can still be a problem in the new formulation – and propofol is often mixed with lidocaine to overcome this (Anon 1998b) – but it could be due to glass fragments (Driscoll *et al.* 1997).

Rate of administration

Rate of administration of intravenous injections and infusions is important. Most anti-emetics are given as a slow intravenous injection to reduce the risk of damage by high concentrations of drug at the site of injection. Most anti-emetics are formulated to an acidic pH. Some of the newer 5-HT_3 antagonists are given as intravenous infusions to further lower the risk of venous irritation.

The directions for the rate of administration suggested in the summary of product characteristics or data sheet for a drug (Anon 1998b) should always be followed by the nurse or anaesthetist giving the drug to prevent unwanted side-effects. At a ward level, the ward pharmacist can endorse the administration directions in the relevant box of the prescription card.

Conclusions

Ideally, all anti-emetics given intravenously should pass through an end-line filter to prevent particulate or microbial contamination from entering the patient. Anti-emetics should only be drawn up immediately before use, or labelled clearly. Anti-emetics should not be mixed with other agents, unless compatibility has been proven. The intravenous route should be used in preference to the intramuscular route for anti-emetic administration, if the oral route is not an option.

Appendix

Cyclizine (Valoid) (Anon 1998b)

Presentation: 50 mg tablets or 50 mg in 1 ml ampoules
Administration: oral, intramuscular or intravenous injection. The intravenous injection should be given slowly, with only minimal withdrawal of blood from the syringe (Anon 1998)
pH: from 3.3 to 3.7 (Trissell 1998)
Stability: cyclizine injection is a colourless solution which should be protected from light. A yellow tint may develop during storage but does not indicate a potency loss. Cyclizine lactate is incompatible with any solution with a pH of 6.8 or greater. Cyclizine has an aqueous solubility of 8 mg/ml. More concentrated solutions may produce crystals within 24 hours (Trissell 1998)
Excipients: none
There has been very little work done on the compatibility of cyclizine with other agents with the exception of agents used in palliative care.
Compatibility (Trissell 1998)
Solution compatibility:

> **Compatible**: glucose 5% and water for injection
> **Incompatible**: sodium chloride 0.9%

Drugs compatible with cyclizine in a syringe for 24 hours:

> **Compatible:** diamorphine (dependent on concentration), diamorphine plus haloperidol (dependent on conc.), haloperidol, morphine (Bradley 1996), methadone (Dhami *et al.* 1995)
> **Incompatible:** probably all drugs containing chloride ions (e.g. metoclopramide, granisetron, ondansetron, tropesetron, chlorpromazine)

Dexamethasone Sodium Phosphate (Anon 1998)

Presentation: 0.5 mg and 2 mg tablets, and 8 mg/2 ml ampoule
Administration: The injection can be given intravenously undiluted over one to several minutes or by continuous or intermittent infusion. It can be also be given by intramuscular injection
pH: from 7 to 8.5
Stability: the ampoules should be protected from light and freezing
Sorption: dexamethasone does not undergo significant absorption in PVC bags or tubing, cellulose burette chambers or in polypropylene or polythene syringes. It is not affected by 5 μm steel filters, 0.22 μm or 0.45 μm cellulose ester membrane or 0.22 μm polycarbonate filters
Excipients: nil
Compatibility (Trissell 1998)
Solution compatibility: dexamethasone is compatible with sodium chloride 0.9% and glucose 5% (see above)

Additive compatibility with dexamethasone:

Compatible: granisetron, ondansetron, prochlorperazine
Incompatible: diphenhydramine plus lorazepam plus metoclopramide

Drugs compatible with dexamethasone in a syringe for 24 hours:

Compatible: granisetron, metoclopramide, ondansetron
Incompatible: not known

Y site injection compatibility with dexamethasone:

Compatible: granisetron, heparin, lorazepam, morphine, ondansetron, pethidine, propofol
Incompatible: ciprofloxacin, midazolam

Droperidol (Droleptan) (Anon 1998b)

Presentation: 10 mg tablets, 1 mg/ml liquid, and 10 mg/2 ml ampoule
Administration: the injection can be given intramuscularly or slow intravenous injection or intermittent or continuous intravenous infusion
pH: from 3 to 3.8
Stability: droperidol should be stored at room temperature and from light
Sorption: there is no problem with droperidol in PVC bags of sodium chloride 0.9% and 5% glucose solution, but sorption does take place in Ringer's solution
Excipients: mannitol, lactic acid
Compatibility (Trissell 1998)
Solution compatibility: droperidol is compatible with sodium chloride 0.9%, glucose 5% solution and Ringer's solution.

Additive compatibility with droperidol:

Compatible: not known
Incompatible: not known

Drugs compatible with droperidol in a syringe for 24 hours:

Compatible: chlorpromazine, fentanyl, metoclopramide, pethidine, midazolam, morphine, nalbuphine, pentazocine, prochlorperazine, promethazine, hyoscine hydrobromide
Incompatible: not known

Y site injection compatibility with droperidol:

Compatible: aztreonam, granisetron, hydrocortisone, metoclopramide, morphine sulphate, potassium chloride, propofol
Incompatible: heparin, tazocin

Granisetron (Kytril) (Anon 1998b)

Presentation: 1 mg and 2 mg tablets, 1 mg/5 ml liquid, and 1 mg/1 ml and 3 mg/1 ml vials
Administration: the injection can be given intravenously after dilution to 1 mg/5 ml over 30 seconds or by intravenous infusion after dilution to 20–50 ml with sodium chloride 0.9% or glucose 5% over five minutes
pH: from 4.7 to 7.3 (Trissell 1998)
Stability: granisetron should be stored at 30°Celsius or less and protected from freezing and light. It is stable to pH changes. It is stable for 24 hours after dilution.
Excipients: none
Compatibility (Trissell 1998)
Solution compatibility: granisetron is compatible with water for injection, sodium chloride 0.9% and glucose 5% solution, sodium chloride 0.18% and glucose 4%, Hartman's solution, sodium lactate infusion, mannitol 10%

Additive compatibility with granisetron:

Compatible: dexamethasone
Incompatible: not known

Drugs compatible with granisetron in a syringe for 24 hours:

Compatible: not known
Incompatible: not known

Y site injection compatibility with granisetron:

Compatible: aztreonam, buprenorphine, most commonly used UK cephalosporins, chlorpromazine, ciprofloxacin, dobutamine, dopamine, droperidol, haloperidol, heparin, hydrocortisone, lorazepam, metoclopramide, metronidazole, morphine sulphate, nalbuphine, pethidine, piperacillin, potassium chloride, prochlorperazine, promethazine, propofol, tazocin, vancomycin
Incompatible: not known

Haloperidol (Anon 1998)

Presentation: 0.5 mg capsules, 1.5 mg, 5 mg, 10 mg and 20 mg tablets, 1 mg/ml and 2 mg/ml liquid, and 5 mg/1 ml, 10 mg/2 ml and 20 mg/2 ml ampoule
Administration: the injection can be given intramuscularly, subcutaneously or by intravenous injection and infusion
pH: from 3 to 3.6
Stability: haloperidol should be stored at room temperature and protected from light. Do not freeze or keep at temperatures above 40° Celsius
Excipients: lactic acid
Compatibility (Trissell 1998)
Solution compatibility: haloperidol is compatible in sodium chloride 0.9% and glucose 5% solution at low concentrations, but incompatible at high concentrations especially in sodium chloride 0.9%.

Additive compatibility with haloperidol:
Compatible: not known
Incompatible: not known

Drugs compatible with haloperidol in a syringe for 24 hours:
Compatible: cyclizine (WFI or glucose 5% solution), diamorphine (dependent on concentration)
Incompatible: ketorolac, morphine

Y site injection compatibility with haloperidol:
Compatible: aztreonam, dobutamine, dopamine, glyceryl trinitrate, granisetron, midazolam, ondansetron, noradrenaline, phenylephrine, propofol
Incompatible: heparin, tazocin

Metoclopramide (Maxolon) (Anon 1998b)

Presentation: 10 mg tablets, 5g/5 ml oral solution, 10 mg/2 ml ampoule, and 100 mg/20 ml vial
Administration: the injection can be given intramuscularly or intravenously undiluted as 10 mg doses over 1 to 2 minutes or by intravenous dilution over 15 minutes after further dilution to 50 ml to 100 ml for larger doses, or to 500 ml and given over 8 to 12 hours
pH: from 3.6 to 6.5
Stability: metoclopramide should be stored at room temperature. It should not be frozen. It is stable over a pH range of 2 to 9. It is also photosensitive, but dilute solutions do not need to be protected from light. Discoloured solutions should be discarded
Excipients: sodium metabisulphite
Compatibility (Trissell 1998)
Solution compatibility: metoclopramide is compatible with most commonly used solutions

Additive compatibility with metoclopramide:

> **Compatible**: morphine sulphate, potassium chloride
> **Incompatible**: erythromycin

Drugs compatible with metoclopramide in a syringe for 24 hours:

> **Compatible**: dexamethasone, diamorphine, droperidol, fentanyl, hyoscine hydrobromide, methotrimeprazine, midazolam, morphine, pentazocine, pethidine, prochlorperazine, promazine, promethazine
> **Incompatible**: not known

Y site injection compatibility with ondansetron:

> **Compatible**: aztreonam, ciprofloxacin, droperidol, granisetron, heparin, morphine sulphate, ondansetron, pethidine, propofol, tazocin
> **Incompatible**: not known

Ondansetron (Zofran) (Anon 1998b)

Presentation: 4 mg and 8 mg tablets, 4 mg/5 ml syrup, 16 mg suppositories and 4 mg/2 ml and 8 mg/4 ml ampoule, 4 mg/2 ml and 8 mg/4 ml plastic (polypropylene) flexi-amps
Administration: the injection can be given intramuscularly or intravenously undiluted over at least 30 seconds and preferably over two to five minutes or over 15 minutes after further dilution with 50 ml of sodium chloride 0.9% or glucose 5%
pH: from 3.3 to 4
Stability: ondansetron is a stable solution. It should be stored at room temperature or refrigerated and protected from light. It is, however, stable for one month in daylight. It is also stable for up to one week when diluted with compatible solutions. Precipitation has been reported if combined with alkaline drugs. Ondansetron is not affected by in line 0.2 μm filters
Excipients: citric acid monohydrate, sodium citrate
Compatibility (Trissell 1998)
Solution compatibility: ondansetron is compatible with most commonly used solutions for up to a week

Additive compatibility with ondansetron:

> **Compatible**: dexamethasone (G5W & NS), morphine sulphate (NS), pethidine (NS)
> **Incompatible**: not known

Drugs compatible with ondansetron in a syringe for 24 hours:

> **Compatible**: dexamethasone (Trissell 1998), alfentanil, atropine, droperidol, fentanyl, glycopyrrolate, metoclopramide, midazolam, morphine, neostigmine, pethidine, and propofol (Stewart *et al.* 1998)
> **Incompatible**: not known

Y site injection compatibility with ondansetron:

> **Compatible**: aztreonam, most commonly used UK cephalosporins, chlorpromazine, dexamethasone, diphenhydramine, droperidol, haloperidol, heparin, hydrocortisone, hydromorphone, metoclopramide, morphine sulphate, pethidine, potassium chloride, prochlorperazine, promethazine, tazocin
> **Incompatible**: ampicillin, lorazepam, piperacillin

Prochlorperazine (Stemetil) (Anon 1998b)

Presentation: prochlorperazine is available as 5 mg and 25 mg tablets, 3 mg buccal tablets, 5 mg/5 ml syrup, 5 mg effervescent sachets, 5 mg and 25 mg suppositories and 12.5 mg/1 ml ampoule
Administration: the injection can be given intramuscularly deep into the upper outer quadrant of the buttock. It can be given undiluted as a slow intravenous injection at a rate not exceeding 5 mg/min to prevent local irritation. An intravenous infusion of 20 mg prochlorperazine per litre of compatible solution is recommended. Subcutaneous injection is not recommended
pH: from 4.2 to 6.2
Stability: intact ampoules can be stored at most temperatures from freezing to 40° Celsius. It should be protected from light, but a slight yellow colour does not reflect loss of potency, however a markedly discoloured solution should be discarded. Prochlorperazine does not undergo significant sorption to a 0.45 μm cellulose membrane filter during infusion
Excipients: sodium sulphite anhydrous (E221), sodium metabisulphite (E223), ethanolamine
Compatibility (Trissell 1998)
Solution compatibility: prochlorperazine is compatible with most commonly used solutions

Additive compatibility with prochlorperazine:

Compatible: dexamethasone (G5W), dimenhydrinate (G5W)
Incompatible: methohexitone (G5W), thiopentone

Drugs compatible with prochlorperazine in a syringe for 24 hours:

Compatible: chlorpromazine, diamorphine, droperidol, fentanyl, hyoscine hydrobromide, metoclopramide, morphine sulphate, nalbuphine, pentazocine, pethidine, promazine, promethazine
Incompatible: ketorolac, midazolam, thiopentone

Y site injection compatibility with prochlorperazine:

Compatible: granisetron, heparin, hydrocortisone, ondansetron, potassium chloride, propofol
Incompatible: aztreonam, tazocin

Promazine (Trissell 1998)

Presentation: promazine is available as 25 mg and 50 mg tablets, 25 mg/5 ml and 50 mg/5 ml oral solution and 50 mg/1 ml ampoule
Administration: The injection can be given by deep intramuscular injection. It can be given diluted as an intravenous injection at a concentration not exceeding 25 mg/ml. Therefore, it cannot be given undiluted. Extravasation should be avoided. It should not be given intra-arterially
pH: from 4 to 5.5
Stability: it should be stored at room temperature. It should be protected from freezing and light. A slight yellow colour does not reflect loss of potency, however a markedly discoloured solution or solutions containing precipitation should be discarded. Promazine can undergo some sorption over a number of hours through some burettes, tubing and PVC bags
Excipients: none
Compatibility (Trissell 1998)
Solution compatibility: Promazine is compatible with most commonly used solutions, but some loss can occur in sodium chloride 0.9% if exposed to light

Additive compatibility with promazine:

Compatible: heparin
Incompatible: methohexitone (G5W & NS), thiopentone (G5W)

Drugs compatible with promazine in a syringe for 24 hours:

Compatible: droperidol, fentanyl, glycopyrrolate, hyoscine hydrobromide, metoclopramide, midazolam, morphine sulphate, pentazocine, pethidine, prochlorperazine, promethazine
Incompatible: not known

Y site injection compatibility with prochlorperazine: no data

Promethazine hydrochloride (Phenergan) (Anon 1998b)

Presentation: promethazine is available as 10 mg and 25 mg tablets, 5 mg/5 ml elixir and 25 mg/1 ml and 50 mg/2 ml ampoule
Administration: the injection can be given by deep intramuscular injection. It can be given undiluted as an intravenous injection into tubing of a running infusion solution at a rate not exceeding 25 mg/min or by slow intravenous injection after diluting to 2.5 mg/ml with water for injection. It can also be given by continuous or intermittent intravenous infusion. Extravasation should be avoided. It should not be given subcutaneously or intra-arterially
pH: from 4 to 5.5
Excipients: sodium sulphite anhydrous (E211), sodium metabisulphite (E223)
Stability: it should be stored at room temperature. It should be protected from freezing and light. It has increasing stability with decreasing pH. Promethazine undergoes significant sorption through silastic sorption but not polyethylene tubing
Compatibility (Trissell 1998)
Solution compatibility: promethazine is compatible with most commonly used solutions

Additive compatibility with promethazine:

Compatible: not known
Incompatible: heparin, methohexitone (G5W), thiopentone

Drugs compatible with promethazine in a syringe for 24 hours:

Compatible: atropine plus pethidine, chlorpromazine, droperidol, fentanyl, glycopyrrolate, hyoscine hydrobromide, metoclopramide, midazolam, morphine sulphate, nalbuphine, pentazocine, pethidine, prochlorperazine, promazine
Incompatible: heparin, ketorolac, thiopentone

Y site injection compatibility with promethazine:

Compatible: aztreonam, ciprofloxacin, granisetron, hydrocortisone, ondansetron, potassium chloride
Incompatible: most cephalosporins, heparin, tazocin

Propofol (Diprivan) (Anon 1998b)

Propofol is an intravenous anaesthetic that has been shown to have anti-emetic properties at its best to be non-emetogenic at its worst. It is included in here for completeness.

Presentation: propofol is a ready to use oil in water emulsion in two concentrations: 1% and 2%. The 1% product is available as 20 ml ampoules, 50 ml and 100 ml vials, 50 ml prefilled syringes. The 2% product is available as a 50 ml prefilled syringe

Administration: Propofol should be well shaken before use. It is usually administered undiluted as an intravenous injection or infusion. It can also be diluted in 5% glucose to a dilution of not less than 2 mg/ml. This is not recommended as propofol is not a preserved product against antimicrobials, and many outbreaks of post-operative infection have occurred. Filters with a pore size less than 5 μm should not be used with propofol because they may restrict the administration and/or cause the breakdown of the emulsion

pH: from 7 to 8.5

Stability: unopened containers should not be kept in a refrigerator, but away from light. Propofol undergoes oxidative generation when exposed to oxygen. Any unused propofol should be discarded 12 hours after spiking the vial. Extreme caution should be taken when adding anything to propofol as it supports microbiological growth. Ideally, no additions should be made, but if any additions are made, they should be done under strict aseptic conditions

Excipients: glycerol, nitrogen, purified egg phosphatide, sodium hydroxide, soybean oil

Compatibility (Trissell 1998)

Drugs compatible with propofol in a syringe for 24 hours:

> **Compatible**: thiopentone
>
> **Incompatible**: not known

Y site injection compatibility with propofol:

> **Compatible**: alfentanil, buprenorphine, chlorpromazine, dexamethasone, droperidol, fentanyl, granisetron, haloperidol, hydromorphone, ketamine, levorphanol, lorazepam, metoclopramide, midazolam, morphine sulphate, nalbuphine, pancuronium, pethidine, sufentanil, vecuronium
>
> **Incompatible**: atracurium, cisatracurium, mivacurium

Tropisetron (Navoban) (Anon 1998b)

Presentation: 5 mg capsules and 5 mg/5 ml ampoules.
Administration: The injection can be given as a slow intravenous injection or into a running infusion or as an intravenous infusion diluted in 100 ml sodium chloride 0.9%
pH: from 5.0 to 5.1 (Georget *et al.* 1997)
Stability: tropisetron should be stored below 25° Celsius. Diluted solutions are stable for up to 24 hours. Diluted solutions are stable for up to three months in PVC or polyolefin bags when stored in a fridge or freezer (Georget *et al.* 1997) or in polyethylene containers or polypropylene syringes for up to two weeks (Brigas *et al.* 1998)
Excipients: not known
Compatibility
Solution compatibility: tropisetron is sodium chloride 0.9%, Ringer's solution, fructose 5% and glucose 5%

Additive compatibility with tropisetron:
Compatible: not known
Incompatible: not known

Drugs compatible with tropisetron in a syringe for 24 hours:
Compatible: not known
Incompatible: not known

Y site injection compatibility with tropisetron:
Compatible: not known
Incompatible: not known

References

Allcutt DA, Lort D & McCullum CN (1983). Final in-line filtration for intravenous infusions: a prospective hospital study. *Br J Surg* **70**, 111–13.

Anon (1993). *The incidence and impact of post-operative nausea* (Glaxo Wellcome, Data on file). Synergy Medical Education, London.

Anon (1998a). *Directory of operating theatres and departments of surgery.* London.

Anon (1998b). *ABPI Compendium of data sheets and summaries of product characteristics 1998–99.* Datapharm Publications Ltd, London.

Aronson JK (1995). Routes of drug administration. 5. Intramuscular injection. *Prescribers J* **35**, 32–6.

Backhouse CM, Ball PR, Booth S *et al.* (1987). Particulate contaminants of intravenous medications and infusions. *J Pharm Pharmacol* **39**, 241–5.

Baumgartner TG, Schmidt GL, Thakker KM *et al.* (1986). Bacterial endotoxin retention by in-line filters. *Am J Hosp Pharm* **43**, 681–4.

Bradley K (1996). Swap data on drug compatibilities. *Pharmacy in Practice* **3**, 69–72.

Brigas F, Sautou-Miranda V, Normand B *et al.* (1998). Compatibility of tropisetron with glass and plastics. Stability under different storage conditions. *J Pharm Pharmacol* **50**, 407–11.

Clayton DG, Shanahan EC, Ordman AJ & Simpson JC (1985). Contamination of the internal jugular cannulae. *Anaesthesia* **40,** 523–8.

Cousins DH & Upton DR (1998). Medication errors. Why we must now act in theatre. *Pharmacy in Practice* **8**, 64–6.

Dann TC (1969). Routine skin preparation before injection: unnecessary procedure. *Lancet* **ii**, 96–8.

De Luca PP, Rapp RP, Bivins BA *et al.* (1976). Filtration and infusion phlebitis: a double blind prospective clinical study. *Am J Hosp Pharm* **33**, 29–34.

Dhami SS, Gahir BS, Hall G & Hall SM (1995). *Pharm J* **255**(6868), R33.

Driscoll DF, Lewis K & Bistrian B (1997). Particle size distribution of propofol injection ampules and vials: the benefits of filtration. *Int J Pharmaceut Compounding* **1**.

Falchuk KH, Peterson L & McNeil BJ (1985). Microparticulate-induced phlebitis: its prevention by in-line filtration. *New Eng J Med* **312**, 78–82.

Francombe P (1998). Intravenous filters and phlebitis. *Nursing Times* **84**, 34–5.

Georget S, Blaise N, Perrin A *et al.* (1997). Stability of refrigerated and frozen solutions of tropisetron in either polyvinylchloride or polyolefin bags. *J Clin Pharm & Ther* **22**, 257–60.

Greenblatt DJ & Allen MD (1978). Intramuscular injection-site complications. *JAMA* **240**, 542–4.

Hipwell CE, Mashford ML & Robertson MB (ed.) (1984). *Guide to parenteral administration of drugs.* ADIS Health Science Press, Sydney.

Holmes CJ, Kundsin RB, Ausman RK & Walter CW (1980). Potential hazards associated with microbial contamination of in-line filters during intravenous therapy. *J Clin Microbiol* **12**, 725–31.

Macmillan EL (1972). Sterile fluids for parenteral infusions. Letter to Secretaries of Hospital Management Committees, 18 August.

Maki DG, Rhame FS, Mackel DC *et al.* (1971). Nosocomial septicaemia subsequent to contaminated intravenous fluid. Presented at the Annual Meeting of the American Society for Microbiology, Minneapolis, 5 May.

Marshall L & Lloyd G (1987). Intravenous fluid filtration. *Care of the Critically Ill* **3**, 10–17.

Ng PC, Herrington RA, Beane CA *et al.* (1989). An outbreak of Acinetobacter septicaemia in a neonatal intensive care unit. *J Hosp Inf* **14**, 363–8.

Quercia RA, Hills SQ, Klimek JJ *et al.* (1986). Bacteriological contamination of intravenous infusion delivery systems in an intensive care unit. *Am J Med* **80**, 364–8.

Sabon RL, Cheung EY, Stommel KA & Hennen CR (1989). Glass particle contamination: influence of aspiration methods and ampule type. *Anesthesiology* **70**, 859–62.

Shaw NJ & Lyall EGH (1985). Hazards of glass ampules. *BMJ* **291**, 1390.

Stewart JT, Warren FT, King DT, Venkateshwaran TG & Fox JL (1998). Stability of ondansetron hydrochloride and 12 medications in plastic syringes. *Am J Health-Syst Pharm* **55**, 2630–4.

Taylor SA (1982). Particulate contamination of sterile syringes and needles. *J Pharm Pharmacol* **34**, 493–5.

Trissell LA (1998). *ASHP handbook on injectable drugs* 10th edn. American Society of Healthcare Pharmacists.

Twum-Danso K, Dawodu AH, Saleh MAF & Makiling LS (1989). An outbreak of Klebsiella pneumoniae bacteraemia in five children on intravenous therapy. *J Hosp Inf* **14**, 271–4.

Uchegbu & Florence (1996). Adverse drug events related to dosage forms and delivery systems. *Drug Safety* **14**(1), 39–67.

Wardle EN (1986). Endotoxins and respiratory and renal failure. *Care of the Critically Ill* **2**, 54–6.

Whipple JK, Quebbeman EJ, Lewis KS *et al.* (1994). Identification of patient controlled analgesia overdose in hospitalised patients: a computerised method of monitoring adverse events. *Ann Pharmacother* **28**, 655–7.

PART 3

Multi-disciplinary approaches and strategies

Chapter 7

Poor clinical outcome from management of PONV: review of theatre-to-ward management following major surgery and hospital-to-home management following day surgery

Andrew Vickers

Introduction

PONV is a distressing though not inevitable sequela of anaesthesia and surgery. It can lead to medical problems such as dehydration, pulmonary aspiration and delayed recovery and discharge. The patient's memory of PONV can be more profound than for pains and the fear of nausea and emesis can be such that patients may refuse analgesics to avoid their side-effects (Orkin 1992).

The aetiology of PONV is complex and multi-factorial; risk factors can be broadly classified as:

- patient characteristics (e.g. predisposition to PONV (previous history) or travel sickness, obesity and the female gender);
- surgical factors (site and duration of surgery, and urgency of procedure);
- anaesthetic factors (e.g. choice of anaesthetic agents, use of opioids);
- post-operative factors (e.g. consumption of opioids, time to oral intake, hypoxia, hypotension and time to ambulation).

Managing PONV

The management of PONV is a multi-modal process and can be considered under the following headings:

- Identifying those patients at risk of PONV
- Use of prophylactic anti-emetics
- Minimising the use of triggering agents during anaesthesia
- Charting of nausea and vomiting scores
- Appropriate prescriptions of anti-emetics
- Prompt treatment of PONV
- Take-home prescriptions of anti-emetics for day-case patients
- Education programmes
- Audit
- Economics

Identifying those patients at risk of PONV

There are many predisposing factors for PONV so priorities should be established to identify those patients most likely to experience it; for example, women with a past history of PONV undergoing major gynaecological surgery should be considered at very high risk, while elderly people having cataract surgery are at low risk. This assessment is important in assuring that those patients at high risk receive prophylactic measures while satisfying financial constraints and minimising side-effects from anti-emetics.

Use of prophylactic anti-emetics and other techniques

Rowbotham (1992) has reviewed randomised controlled trials (RCTs) of prophylactic anti-emetics and concluded that cyclizine, droperidol, prochlorperazine and ondansetron have a prophylactic effect, while the use of metoclopramide is questionable. There are a number of issues which remain unclear, however, such as the optimum dose and ideal time of administration for all of these drugs.

A systematic review of RCTs by Vickers (1996) has demonstrated that acupuncture/acupressure administered before surgery has a prophylactic effect but not if stimulation is performed only during anaesthesia. The use of the P6 point was common to all the studies reviewed. Vickers did comment, however, that the design of all these studies was not ideal and did question his conclusion regarding the efficacy of acupuncture.

Zingiber officinale (ginger root) has been shown to have anti-emetic properties; in a study of women undergoing day case laparoscopy, it was as effective as metoclopramide and superior to placebo in preventing PONV (Phillips 1993).

It is important, however, to remember that *none* of these drugs/methods is totally efficacious.

Minimising triggering agents during anaesthesia

There is conflicting evidence from two systematic reviews (Divatia *et al.* 1996; Tramer *et al.* 1996) whether the omission of nitrous oxide influences the incidence of PONV. All volatile agents are ematogenic, whereas propofol may have significant anti-emetic properties (Watcha *et al.* 1992).

The use of local anaesthetic techniques will reduce opioid requirements both during and after surgery and would be expected to reduce the likelihood of PONV.

The selective use of nasogastric tubes during/after intra-abdominal surgery as opposed to indiscriminate gastric drainage will also help to minimise PONV (Cheatham *et al.* 1995).

Charting of nausea and vomiting scores

Scores for PONV are helpful in highlighting problems and to facilitate audit. The act of recording scores helps focus attention on PONV and, when combined with guidelines for management, will encourage prompt treatment of nausea and/or vomiting.

Appropriate prescriptions of anti-emetics

Anti-emetics fall into three broad groups: the dopamine-2 antagonists, the muscarinic antagonists and the 5-hydroxytryptamine-3 antagonists. Prescriptions for these groups not only should take into account appropriate dose and dosing interval but avoid using two drugs from the same group; if one failed, it is likely that another will do likewise. This is particularly important for the dopamine-2 antagonists where involuntary movement syndromes, such as oculogyric crisis and acute dystonia, can be very distressing consequences of overdose.

Prompt treatment of PONV

It is most important that PONV is recognised and treated promptly. This can only happen if other factors in the process are carried out such as charting PONV scores and prescribing anti-emetics. The use of guidelines may be helpful to ensure this and should necessitate that anti-emetics are used logically for maximum effect and to minimise side-effects. Established PONV should be regarded as a significant complication of surgery and medical and nursing staff should be educated to treat it as such. Failure to institute treatment early can result in other medical complications and patient distress and influence patients' attitudes to future surgery.

Take home anti-emetics for day-case patients

PONV is a significant factor in unexpected overnight stay for day-case patients, but many patients experience PONV only after they have left the hospital. An audit of children undergoing day-case dental extraction in Lancaster demonstrated that more than 25 per cent vomited after leaving hospital. An additional factor in this may be having to endure transport home, which can take up to 60 minutes. The prescription of anti-emetics is complicated by the fact that the patient is not under supervision by medical and nursing staff and side-effects may be significant. A study of low-dose droperidol given prophylactically to day-case patients demonstrated a significant incidence of nightmares for up to 24 hours afterwards. There are no systematic reviews to indicate which medication is best (efficacy versus side-effects) and the optimal dose of any anti-emetic.

Education

Implementation of the process described above is dependent on all the carers involved in the process being aware of PONV and its management. The groups which should be targeted include anaesthetists, non-anaesthetist medical staff and nursing staff. It is unrealistic to assume that knowledge gained at, say, medical school is sufficient and contemporary for this purpose. A regular programme of education should be in place, attendance should be compulsory and written records of attendance kept. Educational programmes can be supported by the use of guidelines to ensure best practice.

Audit

Audit is a valuable tool to examine whether local management of PONV is satisfactory. The incidence of PONV in various patient groups is well established so audit should not be continuous but target specific groups regularly for a fixed period of, say, one week. Appropriate indicators could be the incidence of PONV in that group, the percentage of patients who were prescribed an anti-emetic and the percentage of patients with PONV who received one (Royal College of Anaesthetists 1999).

The Welsh Office (1992) has set standards for PONV with an initial target of no more than 25 per cent of all surgical patients to suffer PONV with the expectation that this would fall to less than 10 per cent but different standards would have to be set for specific groups such as women undergoing major gynaecological surgery.

Economics

Besides being very distressing, PONV also has an economic impact: it may prolong hospital stay, and the cost of treating each emetic episode has been calculated to be approximately £1. Against this must be balanced the use of expensive anti-emetics; the indiscriminate use of these drugs may result in restriction of their use. Once again, the use of guidelines may help to ensure that valuable resources are targeted on those most at risk of PONV (Tang *et al.* 1996).

PONV management – current practices

The factors involved in the optimal management of PONV have been described above but how closely does actual practice match the ideal situation? Is PONV a problem? A review of textbooks will produce a list of options for management but does not describe what is actually done. To try to understand current practice for the management of PONV and why it might fail, a survey was carried out in October/November 1998 of members of the Acute Pain Special Interest Group (APSIG) of the Pain Society. Two hundred and fourteen questionnaires were distributed and 131 were returned and analysed. In considering the results of this survey it must be understood that:

- this is a self-selected group; it is reasonable to assume that anaesthetists or nurses who are motivated to be members of APSIG and the Pain Society are enthusiastic about pain and PONV management and represent the better end of the spectrum of practice;
- it is possible that more than one member of a department is a member of APSIG and so multiple entries from a single department have been received; it is this author's opinion that this will not significantly affect the outcome of the survey.

❑ Have you audited PONV in your hospital?

n=131	Yes	94 (72%)	No	37 (28%)

The responses to this question indicate that some audit has been carried out in many of the departments sampled but do not define how recently this was done, whether audit is recurrent or which groups of patients were targeted.

❑ Do you know the incidence of PONV in your hospital?

n=131	Yes	67 (51%)	No	64 (49%)

Some responses gave an indication of the actual figures for incidence of PONV but this was not specifically sought since the incidence varies so widely between different patient groups.

❑ Do you provide teaching on PONV management to:

New anaesthetists?	Yes	81 (62%)	No	42 (32%)
Other new doctors?	Yes	51 (39%)	No	78 (60%)
Nursing staff?	Yes	85 (65%)	No	44 (34%)

Education for all these groups is the cornerstone of PONV management. The responses to this question indicate that some educational activity is being carried out but, bearing in mind that the population sampled for this survey represents the better end of the spectrum, these results are disappointing. In general terms, the departments which were providing education were also the ones who had guidelines for the management of PONV in place (see below).

All three groups who received training are important links in the chain for providing optimal management of PONV in terms of prophylactic anti-emetics, avoiding triggers and prescribing anti-emetics (anaesthetists), supervising treatment and modifying medication (ward doctors), and charting observations and treating PONV (nurses); ensuring that they understand their responsibilities must be a priority.

❑ Do you have guidelines/policies for the use of anti-emetics in the following situations:

Recovery?	Yes	70 (53%)	No	60 (46%)
Inpatient prophylaxis?	Yes	53 (40%)	No	77 (60%)
Inpatient treatment?	Yes	70 (53%)	No	57 (44%)
Day-case prophylaxis?	Yes	49 (37%)	No	78 (60%)
Day-case take home?	Yes	30 (23%)	No	94 (72%)
Paediatric prophylaxis?	Yes	27 (21%)	No	84 (64%)
Paediatric treatment?	Yes	41 (31%)	No	77 (59%)
Paediatric take home?	Yes	7 (5%)	No	96 (73%)

Some questionnaires had blank responses for one or more of these categories, which accounts for missing percentages. Where a preference was expressed for guidelines or protocols (6 responses), this was always for guidelines.

Guidelines can play a major part in the training of staff. They have an invaluable role in some situations, such as managing rare or life-threatening events, but are very useful also in providing a co-ordinated response to a problem such as PONV which spans a number of different clinical areas and different groups of staff. Guidelines should not be regarded as limiting clinical freedom but encouraging best practice and should be modified in the light of new information and experience (The Royal College of Anaesthetists and The Association of Anaesthetists 1998). Unfortunately, this survey has shown that departments which do not provide comprehensive education programmes do not have guidelines in place either. An example of a guideline for adult PONV can be found in the appendix to this chapter, on page 108.

❑ In your hospital, which of the following drugs are used regularly for (includes multiple responses):

	Prochlorperazine	*Maxolon*	*Droperidol*	*Cyclizine*	*Ondansetron*	*Granisetron*
Prophylaxis	36	62	73	55	77	10
Treatment	104	82	44	101	93	14
Paediatrics	22	30	10	35	53	3
Day case TTO	15	20	4	8	8	2

Dexamethasone is used in two departments for prophylaxis and one for treatment, domperidone is used in five and four respectively and in two departments for children.

Multiple anti-emetics are used in some departments, the most common combinations being cyclizine/ondansetron (11 responses), cyclizine/prochlorperazine (5), cyclizine/droperidol (4) and ondansetron/droperidol (3).

There is wide variation in the drugs used, with most departments employing a variety of different agents. There are some published comparative studies of anti-emetics (Gan *et al.* 1994; Alexander & Fenelly 1997; Fujii *et al.* 1997) which suggest that the 5-HT_3 antagonists ondansetron and granisetron are superior to droperidol and metoclopramide but Tramer *et al.* (1997) in a systematic review of ondansetron in the treatment of *established* PONV failed to show any significant difference between ondansetron, droperidol and metoclopramide. Overall, then, there seems to be insufficient evidence to recommend any particular drug. The use of metoclopramide for prophylaxis is debatable (Rowbotham 1992) as is its use in children in view of the increased risks of involuntary movements such as akathesia. Choice of agents, therefore, should be based on side-effect profile and cost. The 5-HT_3 antagonists have an excellent side-effects profile but are considerably more expensive than either the dopamine-2 antagonists or the antimuscarinics. These costs must be weighed against the suffering and the economic costs of PONV. Granisetron is used in some departments but not as widely as the more established ondansetron; the former has a longer duration of action but is significantly more expensive than ondansetron. The advantages of using an agent with a long duration and minimal side-effects, and avoiding the need for repeat administration may offset the increased costs.

There is very little evidence to guide the use of anti-emetic combinations, although Puejo *et al.* (1996) did show in 100 patients that the combination of droperidol 2.5 mg and ondansetron 4 mg was more effective than either drug alone. The same drugs mixed with morphine in patient-controlled analgesia (PCA) produced a significant reduction in nausea in the first 12 hours after major gynaecological surgery compared to each individual agent (Wrench *et al.* 1996).

❑ Do you regularly mix anti-emetics with analgesics in PCA syringes? If so, which drugs do you commonly use?

n = 131 | Yes 62 (47%) | No 55 (42%)

Droperidol	51
Cyclizine	14
Ondansetron	5
Granisetron	1
Haloperidol	1
Cyclizine/ondansetron	1

There are published data to support the use of anti-emetics in the PCA syringe on efficacy grounds, for example droperidol 0.166 mg/ml added to morphine significantly reduces emetic episodes compared to morphine alone but at the cost of increased sedation (Russell *et al.* 1996). The optimal dose of droperidol which maximises effect while minimising sedation has not been established. The addition of ondansetron to a morphine/droperidol mixture further improves efficacy in the first 12 hours after surgery (Wrench *et al.* 1996). Metoclopramide 0.5 mg/ml mixed with morphine was compared with morphine alone by PCA (Walder & Aitkenhead 1994). The mixture reduced the incidence of moderate to severe nausea but not the overall incidence of nausea.

The addition of anti-emetics to morphine in PCA syringes has a tempting logic; every time the patient receives the triggering agent (morphine) he also receives the 'antidote'. There are some important issues here, though, concerning drug stability, asepsis (especially when many departments buy in sterile preparations of pre-diluted morphine) and the fact that those patients who will not experience distressing PONV must also receive drugs with significant side-effects.

❑ Do you use other techniques for managing PONV?

Acupuncture/acupressure	14
Sea bands	7
Scopaderm (no longer in BNF)	3
Buccastem (prochlorperazine)	2
Reflexology	2
Haloperidol	1
Ginger	1
Inhaled 'Mediswab'	1

The use of acupuncture has been validated but only if it is applied before induction of anaesthesia. It is assumed that 'sea bands' have a similar mechanism of action as acupuncture.

❑ In your hospital do you think PONV is well managed/a problem/no idea?

The questionnaire had two visual analogue scales relating to inpatients and day-cases, respectively. One end of each scale was labelled 'well-managed' and the other 'a problem', a final option was a tick box labelled 'no idea'. There was no intention to submit these results to statistical analysis so, in order to make results clearer, the visual analogue scales were divided into three equal sections which were recorded as 'well managed', 'a problem' and 'a major problem'. The responses to the inpatient question were also assessed in respect of whether the respondent had carried out audit of PONV or not.

	Well managed	*A problem*	*A major problem*	*No idea*
Inpatient	39 (30%)	46 (36%)	37 (29%)	7 (5%)
% who had audited	90%	67%	62%	–
Day case	45 (35%)	32 (25%)	19 (15%)	31 (25%)

There are grounds for optimism here with 30 per cent of respondents feeling that inpatient PONV is well managed and most of these opinions are founded on the basis of audit. In addition one third felt that PONV in day cases is managed well. However, if we bear in mind that this survey reflects the practices and results of well-motivated specialists, there is still room for considerable improvement. Nearly two-thirds of respondents felt that PONV was still a problem in their hospital and the majority had audit evidence for this. The small number of 'no idea' responses for inpatients suggests that most contributors are well aware of the problem of PONV in their hospitals.

The situation for day-cases is less clear with 25 per cent of those questioned having no idea about the incidence of PONV. Audit of day-case patients is more difficult than for inpatients. Postal questionnaires may have a poor response rate and may be biased to those subjects whose experiences have been unpleasant. Telephone follow-up generates a better response rate and should minimise bias but is time-consuming. Despite these reservations, however, one third of respondents felt that PONV was well managed for day cases, and this is a positive finding.

Conclusions

PONV can cause patient distress, medical complications and has financial implications. The aetiology of PONV is multi-factorial and management is a multi-modal process.

A logical approach to the management of PONV is hindered by a dearth of systematic reviews of anti-emetics in terms of optimal dose, dosing intervals, time of administration for prophylaxis and combinations of drugs. Until these are available, management should be based on side-effects and economics with a treatment pathway based on local guidelines.

The practical value of alternative techniques such as acupuncture is unclear.

Teaching the management of PONV should be a priority. It should begin before doctors and nurses have responsibility for patient care and continue throughout their careers. The provision of education programmes in the workplace is time-consuming and must be repeated at regular intervals. It is unrealistic to expect training to be done in spare time, employers should provide recognised time for this both for trainers and trainees. The employment of a specialist nurse in pain and PONV management is an important contribution to this process.

Guidelines should be introduced to encourage best practice. National guidelines should be produced which can be adapted for local use.

Audit should be used to identify problem areas and to assess progress within the local service.

The effective management of PONV remains a problem in many hospitals despite efforts to improve matters.

Appendix

Guideline and algorithm for managing adult PONV

- PONV can cause dehydration and electrolyte imbalance, disrupt surgical wounds, and slow recovery.
- PONV can have many causes, all of which are additive. Try to minimise pain, ensure rest and adequate hydration. Encourage patients to inform staff at an early stage if they feel unwell.
- Try to identify those at most risk of PONV and treat prophylactically for the first 24 hours post-op. – e.g. one drug regularly and another PRN from a different class of drug.
- Anti-emetic drugs are not always effective and may need to be given in combination with H_1 + D_2 antagonists such as cyclizine and prochlorperazine.
- Check the PONV score from the PCA epidural or observation charts, assess 4 hourly or more frequently if indicated.

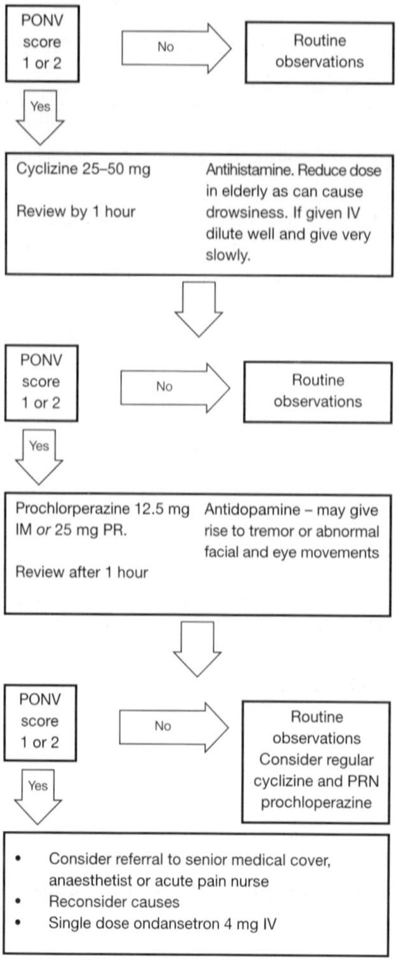

PONV Assessment Score

0 = no nausea or vomiting
1 = nausea or vomiting x 1
2 = severe nausea and vomiting > 1
X = anti-emetic given

Risk Factors

- Emergency surgery
- Major abdominal surgery
- Gynaecology, ENT and eye surgery
- Previous history of PONV
- Post-operative ileus
- Obesity
- Women more so than men
- History of travel sickness
- Anxiety and distress
- Planned early mobilisation
- Low blood pressure

Other anti-emetic therapies

- Ondansetron 5-HT_3 inhibitor, used mainly for nausea associated with chemotherapy. May cause headache or flushing.
- Metoclopramide dopamine and 5-HT_3 antagonist. Least effective anti-emetic (no better than placebo in some trials) but can relieve full feeling in stomach. Not to be used after upper GI or gastric surgery.

Management of anti-emetic side-effects

- Extrapyramidal effects such as tremor, dystonia – particularly of the head and neck and abnormal eye movements – can be reversed by giving 1–2 mg of Benztropine given IM or IV (0.5–1 mg in the elderly)

References

Alexander R, Fenelly M (1997). Comparison of ondansetron, metoclopramide and placebo as premedicants to reduce nausea and vomiting after major surgery. *Anaesthesia* **52**, 695–8.

Cheatham M, Chapman W, Key S, Sawyers J (1995). A meta-analysis of selective versus routine nasogastric decompression after elective laparotomy. *Annals of Surgery* **221**, 469–78.

Divatia J, Vaidya J, Badwe R, Hawaldar R (1996). Omission of nitrous oxide during anaesthesia reduces the incidence of postoperative nausea and vomiting – a meta-analysis. *Anesthesiology* **85**, 1055–62.

Fujii-Y, Toyooka-H, Tanaka-H (1997). Prevention of postoperative nausea and vomiting with granisetron, droperidol and metoclopramide in female patients with a history of motion sickness. *Canadian Journal of Anaesthesia* **44**, 820–4.

Gan T, Collis R, Hetreed M (1994). Double-blind comparison of ondansetron, droperidol and saline in the prevention of postoperative nausea and vomiting. *BJA* **72**, 544–7.

Orkin F (1992). *Anaesthesia & Analgesia* **74**, S225.

Phillips S, Ruggier R & Hutchinson S (1993). Zingiber officinale (ginger) – an antiemetic for day case surgery. *Anaesthesia* **48**, 715–17.

Pueyo F, Carrascosa F, Lopez L, Iribarrau M, Garcia Pedrajas F & Saez A (1996). Combination of ondansetron and droperidol in the prophylaxis of postoperative nausea and vomiting. *Anesth Analg* **83**(1), 117–22.

Rowbotham D (1992). Current management of postoperative nausea and vomiting. *British Journal of Anaesthesia* **69**(Suppl.1), S46–S59.

The Royal College of Anaesthetists and The Association of Anaesthetists (1998). *Good practice – a guide for departments of anaesthesia.* RCA, London.

The Royal College of Anaesthetists (1996). *Audit recipe book* (in press). RCA, London.

Russell D, Duncan L, Frame W, Higgins S, Asbury A & Millar K. Patient controlled analgesia with morphine and droperidol following caesarian section under spinal anaesthesia. *Acta Anaesthesiologica Scand* **40**, 600–5.

Tang J, Watcha M & White P (1996). A comparison of costs and efficacy of ondansetron and droperidol as prophylactic antiemetic treatment for elective gyneacological surgery. *Anesthesia and Analgesia* **83**, 304–13.

Tramer M, Moore A & McQuay H (1996). Omitting nitrous oxide in general anaesthesia: meta-analysis of intraoperative awareness and postoperative emesis in randomized controlled trials. *British Journal of Anaesthesia* **76**, 186–93

Tramer M, Moore A, Reynolds D & McQuay H (1997). A qualitative systematic review of ondansetron in the treatment of established postoperative nausea and vomiting. *BMJ* **314**, 1088–92.

Vickers A (1996). Can acupuncture have specific effects on health? A systematic review of acupuncture antiemesis trials. *Journal of the Royal Society of Medicine* **89**, 303–11.

Walder A & Aitkenhead A (1994). Antiemetic efficacy of metoclopramide when included in a patient-controlled analgesia infusion. *Anaesthesia* **49**, 804–6.

Watcha M & White P (1992). Postoperative nausea and vomiting – its etiology, treatment and prevention. *Anesthesiology* **77**, 162–84.

The Welsh Office (1992). Welsh Health Planning Forum.

Wrench I, Ward J, Walder A, Hobbs G (1996). The prevention of postoperative nausea and vomiting using a combination of ondansetron and droperidol. *Anaesthesia* **51**, 776–8.

Acknowledgments

The author would like to thank Dr Malvena Stuart Taylor for her suggestions for audit indicators and Dr David Counsell, of Victoria Hospital, Blackpool, for his algorithm for managing PONV.

Chapter 8

Improving clinical outcome from management of PONV: the developing role of the anaesthetist, pharmacist and multi-disciplinary team

Fiona Dobson, Steve Haigh & Greg Hobbs

Introduction

Current outcomes from the management of PONV are far from acceptable. This is partly the result of poor organisation and insufficient emphasis on proper medical and nursing priorities in the delivery of peri-operative care. There is also a delay in getting research evidence into practice. It is unrealistic to expect significantly improved outcomes without a new, multi-disciplinary strategy to reorganise PONV management. The contributions of anaesthetists, pharmacists and nursing staff are crucial to this strategy. Their roles are examined below.

The developing role of the anaesthetist

Current practice, current roles

The current management of PONV has two components: prevention and treatment. Prevention has largely been the domain of the anaesthetist. Published research, the bulk performed by clinical and academic anaesthetists, has quantified risk prediction (Toner *et al.* 1996) and demonstrated that single anti-emetic prophylaxis reduces the incidence and severity of PONV (although at best the reduction is about 50 per cent). Anaesthetists undertaking good clinical practice make an informal review of PONV risk during their pre-operative patient assessment, commonly give a single prophylactic anti-emetic during surgery if the patient is considered to be 'at risk' and write the prescription, usually a single anti-emetic, for the post-operative treatment of PONV. The treatment of established PONV is traditionally managed by ward doctors and nursing staff. This disparate clinical process continues to be associated with an incidence of PONV of about 25 per cent (Watcha & White 1992; Koivuranta *et al.* 1997).

What needs to change?

It should be obvious that both the current organisation and clinical process for managing PONV are ineffective. There are a number of contributing factors which point to potential roles for the anaesthetist.

The management of research

PONV research usually evaluates pharmacological interventions. Recent evidence of the high efficacy of combination anti-emetic prophylaxis (see Chapter 5) suggests that outcomes can be significantly improved. So why does proven efficacy fail to improve clinical effectiveness? Strategies to improve outcomes in clinical practice have not been addressed. Research should take a more pragmatic direction and evaluate daily practice and whole clinical regimens or packages. There is a need to get strategy into research as well as research into strategy.

The wrong perspective? No incentive or resources for change

The process for managing PONV is influenced strongly by a medical perspective. Medical staff, unlike nursing professionals, usually have little involvement with the direct consequences of PONV. This albeit-justified isolation of medicine discourages anaesthetists' interest in contributing to changing practice. However, patients often rate PONV as their most distressing post-operative experience. Achieving humanitarian outcomes is a primary consideration for the improvement of peri-operative care.

The management of PONV lacks glamour. PONV is neither a critical incident nor major morbidity. Without a reputation for 'seriousness', PONV attracts scant interest from professionals who control the resources available for peri-operative care. Other than existing expenditure on anti-emetic drugs and relevant disposables, there are no specific resources or budget dedicated to the management of PONV.

Knowledge, attitudes and expectations

Mismatched expectations of outcomes by patients and staff alike do not facilitate change. We have been able to demonstrate changes in patient expectation in acute pain management using an interactive nursing approach to delivering patient information; this should also be possible in PONV management. Training of anaesthetists and other doctors may improve the use of intra-operative prophylaxis and post-operative prescribing, but without education of nursing staff and patients there is no guarantee that an appropriate anti-emetic prescription will be used effectively, if at all.

A lack of information

Few anaesthetists, ward staff or patients will have an accurate knowledge of the incidence of PONV in their area of work. There is usually little local examination of process and outcomes from PONV management other than isolated audit projects. Are patients adequately assessed for risk of PONV and is prophylaxis used appropriately? Have all post-operative patients an evidence-based anti-emetic prescription available and how is it used? Without a continuous audit programme and appropriate dissemination of results there will be neither appreciation of the need for change nor ammunition to bring about such change.

Roles, goals and accountability

All professionals and patients should be aware of their roles and responsibilities in the process of managing PONV. This is unlikely without intensive education and training both inside and outside the theatre environment. We know of few other hospitals with explicit goals or standards for outcomes from PONV management. Who is accountable for these basic humanitarian outcomes in your hospital?

No strategy, no change

Sustained, local improvement in outcomes from PONV may well need widespread, permanent changes to clinical practice both in the traditional anaesthetic environment and on hospital wards. An effective strategy for improving outcomes from PONV must examine pre-operative, intra-operative and post-operative care relevant to the management of PONV.

Momentum for change

Momentum for change can now be identified readily in the professional environment of the anaesthetist.

The local environment

There may be local audit and research findings and motivated professionals who are interested in improving outcomes. This interest and evidence will be useful for promoting recognition of the need for change.

The external environment

Clinical governance has been given a high priority in the NHS (Department of Health 1998). The report of the Audit Commission (1997) *Anaesthesia under Examination*, and the publication *Good Practice* by the Royal College of Anaesthetists and the Association of Anaesthetists of Great Britain and Ireland (1998) provide valuable sources of advice and recommendations to help negotiate change. *The Anaesthesia Team* from the Association of Anaesthetists of Great Britain and Ireland (1998) promotes the concept of multi-disciplinary working in peri-operative care.

Improving outcomes

The NHS 'drive for quality' provides an opportunity for anaesthetists to develop their roles in improving PONV outcomes.

Leadership

A lack of effective leadership is a major factor contributing to poor outcomes. An effective leader needs ability as an entrepreneur and negotiator of change in a multi-disciplinary setting. An individual should be identified and given responsibility for reorganising strategy for PONV management in each hospital. The ability to set up or use an existing structure to deliver this strategy into practice at all levels of peri-operative care will be the crucial test of effectiveness. Identifying and nurturing appropriate nursing leadership and pharmacy skills will enhance effectiveness.

Developing and implementing a new strategy

Our experience in service development suggests that strategy should give priority to the following elements:

- *Define quality and good practice.* Consider perspectives of patients and all professionals involved in peri-operative care. Acceptability, access to appropriate knowledge, skill, anaesthetic technique and anti-emetic therapy, timeliness of care and costs are all components of 'quality'. PONV must join the key indicators of the quality of peri-operative care.

- *Get serious about audit.* In the absence of dedicated resources to undertake audit, the process can be built into existing care. Information and therefore audit are fundamental to effective change (Jones & McDonnell 1993). While irksome, documenting actual clinical practice as well as its outcomes returns a rapid yield.

- *Facilitate education.* Knowledge, attitudes and expectations of patients and professionals must be geared to maximise effectiveness. Individuals' roles and responsibilities in care must be clear before the event.

- *Use clinical guidelines.* Guidelines can change practice, improve patient care and reduce costs (Busch *et al.* 1998; Nolte *et al.* 1998). However, there is a problem getting them executed effectively. Therefore, guidelines must be *implemented* (and not just disseminated) using rigorous education and monitoring. Team working may be a key factor in the effectiveness of guidelines (McNicol *et al.* 1993). Such models for introducing clinical guidelines and reducing inconsistencies in practice are available. The acute pain service (Commission on the Provision of Surgical Services 1990) and the integrated care pathway are examples (Campbell *et al.* 1998).

Is it worth the investment?

Changing the management of PONV will make new demands on the time of those providing leadership and implementation. There may be challenges from professionals who prioritise absolute personal clinical freedom. However, there is momentum for change, encouraging new research findings and a great opportunity to improve patient and staff outcomes from PONV. Effective change is also likely to enhance the professional development of anaesthetists and other professionals, the reputation of the anaesthetic community and hospital. The challenge to anaesthetists is to contribute to effective leadership; a key, developing role for improving outcomes.

The developing role of the pharmacist

Historically, pharmacists were employed mainly in manufacturing and dispensing roles. These activities have now been delegated on a large scale to more appropriately qualified staff, thus releasing time for hospital pharmacists to be more involved with the promotion of safe, effective and economic use of medicines, in particular at ward level (Hawkey *et al.* 1990). Pharmacists have extensive experience in evaluating the clinical and economic aspects of therapeutic regimens and the development of clinical guidelines. As current management of PONV relies heavily on drug therapy, pharmacists can make important contributions to the choice, implementation and monitoring of therapeutic strategies.

A source of information

The published literature contains an overwhelming amount of data on anti-emetic drugs. (A Medline search of five commonly used anti-emetics reveals over 8,000 papers.) These studies vary in both quality and relevance, and critical appraisal is essential to ensure that decision making about drug use is based on objective evidence of quality. Drug information pharmacists, located in most hospitals, have easy access to a variety of medical, pharmacy and nursing databases and are experienced in reviewing the literature on a regular basis. Pharmacists have a key role in setting up and maintaining the evidence base for use in the management of PONV.

Changing drug use

Developing and implementing guidelines for the use of drugs by medical and nursing staff are never as straightforward as one would hope. Other groups invariably become involved when changes to drug use are expected, particularly when an additional cost is anticipated. Such groups rightly include drug and therapeutic committees, who oversee the use of drugs within hospitals, and budget holders, who must pay the bill. Consulting these groups is mandatory in order for good proposals to be accepted and to maximise the effectiveness and speed of change which reduces PONV; pharmacists are well placed to co-ordinate these activities.

Pharmacoeconomic evaluation

The spending of public funds necessitates proper evaluation of therapeutic choices. Pharmacoeconomics is the science of maximising value for money from health care, using rational, evidence-based decision making. (See Drummond *et al.* (1997) for further details.) Many pharmacists have developed skills in pharmacoeconomic evaluation which are highly relevant to surgical care. For example, the decision about which anti-emetic regimen is most acceptable for inclusion in prescribing guidelines will consider not only the evidence for efficacy but also the associated clinical and economic costs. These aspects will differ between hospitals according to the types of surgery and local drug-purchasing arrangements. Further, nursing and patient perspectives are necessary considerations when developing prescribing guidelines. For example, the choice of an anti-emetic with an intravenous formulation and licence may enhance nursing practice and patients' perception of care compared to the use of intramuscular injections. Thorough pharmacoeconomic evaluations consider all of these factors and provide an estimate of the likely clinical and economic impact of a change to practice. Local data are likely to add relevance to data from the literature in such an evaluation.

Education and monitoring

The drug prescription charts of nearly all patients in hospitals are scanned daily by pharmacists. This intensive monitoring makes a key contribution to risk management in hospital wards (Hawkey *et al.* 1990) and gives an opportunity to evaluate and collect data on outcomes from changes in practice. For example, the effect of introducing new prescribing guidelines can be evaluated at the point of delivery of care with deviations from expected practice detected and rectified by informal guidance and advice at an early stage, often on a one-to-one supervisory basis.

Pharmacy information systems can produce detailed, hospital-wide information on the use and costs of drugs such as anti-emetics. These data can be used to evaluate not only the effect of prescribing recommendations but also give a pre-audit indication of probable clinical outcomes. The pharmacy network can therefore provide a more continuous and realistic picture of practice outcomes than the impressions of clinical staff who have an intermittent presence on wards and who are primarily focused on each individual patient's care.

Pharmacists have a great deal of experience in optimising the use of drugs in hospitals. This experience is readily available in the development and implementation of changes to prescribing practice.

Developing a multi-disciplinary team approach to the reduction of PONV

Is PONV a multi-disciplinary problem?

Viewed simplistically it is easy to assume that PONV is merely a temporary inconvenience for the patient and for the staff directly involved in managing the problem, namely recovery room and ward nursing staff. More extensive analysis reveals PONV to be complex and multi-factorial, influenced by considerations including pre-operative patient preparation, individual patient risk factors, intra-operative interventions and post-operative management techniques. It is therefore not surprising that PONV in adults has remained at a consistent rate of 25 per cent (Watcha & White 1992) and that dependence on post-operative intervention by recovery room and ward nursing staff has failed to reduce this level of incidence.

Further reductions in the incidence of PONV can be achieved by improved pharmacological prophylaxis, less emetogenic anaesthetic techniques, better pain and anti-emesis management and less invasive surgical procedures (Wilder-Smith *et al.* 1993). This is dependent on the implementation of a range of measures by various members of the multi-disciplinary team and will only be achieved if the relevant personnel are aware of the problem, have the necessary resources available to them and the knowledge to select and apply them appropriately.

Multi-disciplinary anti-emesis teams – extravagance or necessity?

Described as the 'big little problem' (Fisher 1997), PONV holds a position of low significance in the overall scheme of surgical management and as such is unlikely to attract specific funding to enable the establishment of a team with the definitive remit of reducing its incidence. This is neither necessary nor sufficient. More than half the hospitals in the UK already have well-established acute pain teams (Audit Commission 1997) or have adopted alternative approaches to dealing with the multi-disciplinary issue of pain management by initiating pain management groups or devolving responsibility for change to a designated existing group such as a practice development group. Providing such groups have multi-professional representation, there is no reason to create a further specialist team.

At Queen's Medical Centre, the acute pain service has assumed responsibility for monitoring and reducing the incidence of PONV. Some might view this work as just deserts, since pain and its management with opioids, particularly via patient-controlled analgesia pumps, are so frequently cited as causative agents.

The role of the acute pain service

PONV and post-operative pain have a striking number of similarities:

- their occurrence is common and unpleasant;
- they are multi-factorial in nature and have implications for post-operative morbidity and prolongation of hospital stay;
- they can both be improved by changing peri-operative management strategies;
- drug therapy is a current keystone to their combined management;
- successful amelioration is dependent upon engaging a large number of health care workers from a range of professions in the adoption and maintenance of changes to their normal practice.

The acute pain service catalyses this process by reviewing existing outcomes, identifying areas for improvement, developing comprehensive management tools, supporting their introduction through education programmes and evaluating the results.

Reviewing the *status quo*

Clinical audit provides an excellent means of determining existing practice and outcomes and targeting areas for change. The specialist nurses within our acute pain service assume responsibility for co-ordinating audits within clinical areas, in consultation with relevant clinical directors and ward nursing colleagues and there is a well-established programme of audit which monitors pain assessment, pain and PONV management outcomes and patient satisfaction.

Involving medical and ward nursing colleagues in developing audit tools is crucial since it offers them ownership of the information and provides a forum for identifying specific problem issues within their own specialties. Collecting data is usually undertaken by acute pain service specialist nurses with support from either the ward's pain link nurse, a ward/department nurse specifically designated to the project or by a research/audit nurse seconded from the particular clinical area to the acute pain service for a defined time period.

Following data collection and analysis, the results plus recommendations for change are presented to the clinical director and senior nurse for their information and agreement. Any changes to recommendations are made at this stage since their support will influence overall compliance with change. Finally data, recommendations and the agreed change strategy are presented to all relevant personnel. Active involvement of clinical colleagues at all stages in the audit process has been demonstrated to be superior to the unsolicited provision of information with no stated action plan (Mugford *et al.* 1991; Thomson *et al.* 1998).

The *status quo* in relation to PONV

About three years ago we attempted to improve the management of PONV by implementing:

- a set of guidelines for prevention;
- a protocol for treatment of PONV.

The guidelines were directed toward anaesthetists and recommended the use of prophylactic intravenous cyclizine in patients with risk factors for PONV. The protocol focused attention on better prescribing of anti-emetics for the treatment of established PONV through the use of pre-printed anti-emetic prescription labels (Figure 8.1). Nursing colleagues in recovery rooms and on wards were encouraged to monitor PONV more closely, with the anti-emetic prescription protocol giving them the

QMC	**Adult Anti-Emetic Prescription** (If nausea persists 30 minutes after Cyclizine → Ondansetron and continue Cyclizine 8 hrly prn)										
Acute	Cyclizine	Date					Ondansetron	Date			Signed ________
Pain	50 mg iv/im	Time					4 mg iv/im	Time			
Service	8 hrly prn	Route					4 hrly x 2 only	Route			
		Given						Given			Date / /

(*Source:* Queen's Medical Centre, Nottingham)

Figure 8.1 Pre-printed anti-emetic prescription label

opportunity to administer doses of two different anti-emetics within 30 minutes of each other, if appropriate.

Extensive audit demonstrated a significant increase (from approximately 20 to 40 per cent) in the number of patients receiving prophylaxis and a significant change in prophylactic anti-emetic given to cyclizine. Use of the prescription labels by anaesthetists increased the availability of two anti-emetics for treating PONV from 3 to 80 per cent of patients. There were clinical improvements associated with these clear changes in anti-emetic prescription and administration, including a reduction from 30 to 22 per cent in the number of patients recording moderate or severe nausea in the first 24 hours after surgery. A similar reduction in the number of patients receiving anti-emetics on wards (despite more reliable nursing access to appropriate anti-emetic prescriptions) suggested that this change was the result of better prophylaxis and treatment in operating theatres. However, subsequent audits carried out in general surgery, orthopaedics, gynaecology and ENT patients in 1998 all demonstrated an ongoing problem with PONV. The overall incidence during the first 12–48 hours post-operatively persists at around 25 per cent. Further, there has been some 'drift' in the choice of anti-emetic for prophylaxis with cost implications for the anaesthetic drug budget.

Developing a framework for change

The acute pain service decided to address this problem by incorporating the existing guidelines and PONV treatment protocol into a comprehensive PONV management strategy. A proposal was submitted to and approved by the local ethics committee, the key aims of the project being to develop a comprehensive management tool to improve PONV outcomes for patients and staff and to evaluate it.

Specific clinical areas were identified for participation in the project, namely the operating department, recovery room and two gynaecology wards. The project was divided into three phases:

- Clinical audit of at least 100 patients to establish current standards of management and to determine patients' expectations, beliefs and preferences in relation to PONV.

- Development of the management tool and supporting documentation including:
    - a patient information leaflet
    - information/educational tools for theatre and ward nursing/medical staff
    - a nurse-led PONV risk assessment tool
    - anti-emetic prescribing guidelines
    - a patient satisfaction tool for regular use in everyday clinical practice
    - education of all staff involved in implementing the change
    - implementation of the management tool and supporting processes.
- Second clinical audit of at least 100 patients to evaluate the effects of the management changes.

Two staff nurses from the gynaecology wards were seconded part time to the acute pain service for one year. They are fully involved in all data collection and analysis, developing the required documentation and participating in the education programme. Most importantly, because they are still working on their wards, they can act as opinion leaders influencing the rate of uptake of change by ward nursing and medical colleagues (Bury 1998).

It is impractical to assume that specialist nurses within an acute pain service can take direct responsibility for the management of PONV: at Queen's Medical Centre this would necessitate visits to around 40,000 patients each year. Neither is this approach desirable. One of the criticisms frequently levelled at specialist nurses is that they deskill nursing colleagues by taking over specific elements of care (Humphris 1994). As with pain management, our approach necessitates increasing the skills of colleagues, giving them the knowledge, authority, confidence and support to function autonomously within the multi-disciplinary team – an issue which is critical in terms of changing practice and improving patient outcomes (Fulton 1997).

There are a number of other reasons for identifying ward nurses as key players:

- they represent a relatively stable population of the ward workforce;
- they are directly exposed, on a daily basis, to patients with pain and nausea;
- they are typically involved in pre-admission unit patient assessments;
- they have 24-hour responsibility for pre- and post-operative patient management, including pain and PONV monitoring;
- they have a vested interest in improving pain and PONV management since these problems have a direct impact on their workload and the suffering they see.

Implementing the framework

A preliminary audit of 140 patients stratified into operation types was completed and these data are currently being used to develop the documentation required in the second phase of the project. Examples of the patient information leaflet and management tool are given (Figures 8.2 and 8.3) but are yet to be validated through consultation with patients and peers.

Acute Pain Service

SICKNESS AFTER SURGERY

Some people worry about feeling or being sick after an operation. This leaflet answers the questions that patients often ask.

Q. Is everyone sick after an operation?
A. No. Roughly one third of people feel sick, whilst two thirds usually don't.

Q. Are some people more likely to be sick than others?
A. Some people seem more sensitive to treatments than others. Also how long the operation takes, the sort of operation it is and which pain killers are used can have an effect.

Q. Can sickness be prevented?
A. Yes. There are drugs which can be given at the same time as the anaesthetic. It is important to tell the nurse or the anaesthetist of any worries you have. Before your operation they will ask you questions to see if you are more likely than usual to feel sick.

Q. Is it necessary to have an injection?
A. Not usually. We use a special needle for your anaesthetic which we leave in the back of your hand or arm to save jabbing you again.

Q. How long does the feeling of sickness last?
A. Everybody is different. Usually sickness soon passes off, especially once some treatment has been given.

Q. Can I do anything to avoid feeling sick?
A. Yes. After your operation try not to make sudden movements. When sitting up or getting out of bed, move slowly and smoothly.

When you start drinking take small sips and build up to proper drinking gradually. Eat small light meals to start with.

If you do feel sick, take slow deep breaths to reduce the sensation. Most importantly, tell a nurse as soon as you feel the slightest bit sick.

SIX TOP TIPS FOR COPING WITH SICKNESS

- Warn us if you've felt sick after other operations
- Tell a nurse straight away if you feel sick
- Move slowly and smoothly
- Drink small sips to begin with
- Eat little, light and often
- Try taking deep breaths if sickness strikes

REMEMBER

The staff at QMC understand how unpleasant it is to feel sick. We will do everything to prevent it. If you are unfortunate enough to suffer any sickness we will treat you promptly and give you privacy and support.

Developed for QMC patients with the help of QMC patients

Source: Queen's Medical Centre, Nottingham

Figure 8.2 Patient PONV information leaflet

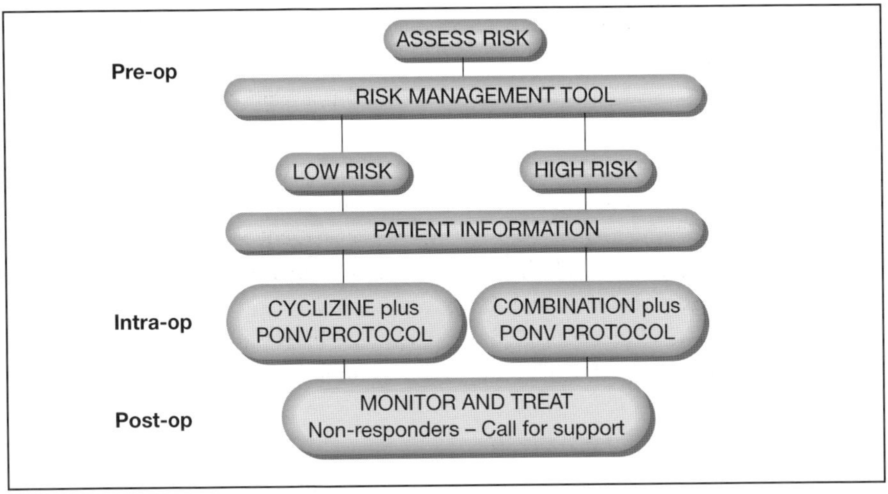

Source: Queen's Medical Centre, Nottingham

Figure 8.3 PONV management tool

Once the necessary documentation has been agreed, a comprehensive education programme will be delivered targeting *all* key personnel. The programme will be tailored to each professional group since their information needs and individual roles are well defined within the strategy (see Box 8.1).

Ensuring that all relevant personnel have the necessary information requires a major investment in time and input from all members of the multi-disciplinary acute pain service. In particular, it is beneficial if nurses speak to nurses and the professions allied to medicine, and doctors to doctors. This class-structured approach is firmly grounded in the realities of professional credibility and opinion leadership (Bury 1998) and shared values and approaches to practice (Pietroni *et al.* 1994).

Box 8.1

- ❑ Gynaecology ward nurses will undertake pre-operative risk assessment, identify high-risk patients, educate patients pre-operatively and support this with the information leaflet, continue to monitor PONV and implement the existing PONV treatment protocol, refer on non-responders.
- ❑ Anaesthetists will reinforce information given by ward nurses, give prophylactic single or combination anti-emetic therapy according to identified risk, continue to prescribe according to the PONV protocol, act as an information resource and medical support for ward colleagues.
- ❑ Operating department practitioners and anaesthetic nurses will support and re-inforce the implementation of the strategy with anaesthetist colleagues.
- ❑ Recovery room nurses will reinforce information given by ward nurses, continue to monitor PONV and implement the PONV treatment protocol.
- ❑ Ward-based medical staff will support the strategy by maintaining appropriate prescriptions for anti-emetics, refer on non-responders.
- ❑ Physiotherapists will inform ward nurses if patients are unable to comply with therapy because of PONV.
- ❑ Acute pain service specialist nurses will attend non-responders and implement alternative strategies for the management of PONV, seek anaesthetist advice in this process when necessary, support all staff through the change process.

Conclusions

The complex nature of PONV suggests that a comprehensive multi-disciplinary team approach to its management is more likely to prove successful than single-profession unilateral interventions. An acute pain service with experience of clinical audit, implementation of change and management of pain and side-effect problems, including PONV, is ideally placed to provide the knowledge, expertise and impetus for improving practice. In the absence of a mature acute pain service, an alternative multi-disciplinary vehicle with roles in peri-operative care could be used to deliver the necessary changes to practice.

Development of an extensive PONV management strategy should be strongly influenced by patients and representatives of those professional groups capable of influencing PONV outcomes. Ward nurses and anaesthetists occupy fundamental positions within this process, but success requires able support by a number of other key professionals.

References

The Association of Anaesthetists of Great Britain and Ireland (1998). *The anaesthesia team.*

Audit Commission (1997). *Anaesthesia under examination.* Audit Commission Publications, Abingdon.

Bury T (1998). Getting research into practice. In *Evidence-based healthcare: a practical guide for therapists* (ed. T Bury & J Mead). Butterworth Heinemann, Oxford.

Busch AF, Pearce MJ, Allen B *et al.* (1996). Compliance with guidelines results in appropriate ondansetron prescribing at Christchurch Hospital. *NZ Med J* **109**, 142–4.

Campbell H, Hotchkiss R, Bradshaw N *et al.* (1998). Integrated care pathways. *BMJ* **316**, 133–7.

Commission on the Provision of Surgical Services (1990). *Report of the Working Party on Pain After Surgery.* Royal College of Surgeons of England, London.

Department of Health (1998). *A first class service. Quality in the new NHS.* The Stationery Office, London.

Drummond MF, O'Brien B, Stoddart *et al.* (1997). *Methods for the economic evaluation of healthcare programmes* 2nd edn. Oxford University Press, Oxford.

Fisher DM (1997). The 'big little problem' of postoperative nausea and vomiting (Editorial). *Anesthesiology* **87**, 1271–2.

Fulton Y (1997). Nurses' views on empowerment: a critical social theory perspective. *J Adv Nurs* **26**, 529–36.

Hawkey C J *et al.* (1990). Effect of reactive pharmacy intervention on quality of hospital prescribing. *BMJ* **300**, 986–90.

Humphris D (1994). *The clinical nurse specialist: issues in practice.* MacMillan Press, Basingstoke.

Jones A & McDonnell U (1993). *Managing the clinical resource.* Bailliere Tindall, London.

Koivuranta M, Laara E, Snare L *et al.* (1997). A survey of postoperative nausea and vomiting. *Anaesthesia* **52**, 443–9.

McNicol M, Layton A & Morgan G (1993). Team working: the key to implementing guidelines? *Quality in Health Care* **2**, 215–16.

Mugford M, Banfield P & O'Hanlon M (1991). Effects of feedback of information on clinical practice: a review. *BMJ* **303**, 398–402.

Nolte MJ, Berkery R, Pizzo B *et al.* (1998). Assuring the optimal use of serotonin antagonist anti-emetics: the process for development and implementation of institutional anti-emetic guidelines at Memorial Sloan-Kettering Cancer Center. *J Clin Oncol* **16**, 771–8.

Pietroni P (1994). Inter-professional teamwork. Its history and development in hospitals, general practice and community care (UK). In *Going inter-professional: working together for health and welfare* (ed. A Leathard). Routledge, London.

The Royal College of Anaesthetists and The Association of Anaesthetists of Great Britain and Ireland (1998). *Good practice. A guide for departments of anaesthesia.* RCA, London.

Thomson MA, Oxman AD, Davis DA *et al.* (1998). Audit and feedback to improve health professional practice and health care outcomes (part II). In *Cochrane Collaboration on Effective Professional Practice Module of the Cochrane Database of Systematic Reviews* (ed. L Bero, R Grilli, J Grimshaw *et al.*). Update Software, Oxford.

Toner CC, Broomhead IH, Littlejohn GS *et al.* (1996). Prediction of postoperative nausea and vomiting using a logistic regression model. *British Journal of Anaesthesia* **76**, 347–51.

Watcha MF & White PF (1992). Postoperative nausea and vomiting: its etiology, treatment and prevention. *Anesthesiology* **77**, 162–84.

Wilder-Smith OHG, Martin NC & Morabia A (1993). Postoperative nausea and vomiting: a comparative survey of the attitudes, perceptions and practice of Swiss anesthesiologists and surgeons. *Anesthesia and Analgesia* **84**, 826–31.

Postscript

Since the preparation of this chapter, the project to develop and evaluate the comprehensive management tool to improve PONV outcomes in gynaecological wards (Figure 8.3) has been completed. The results suggest that the use of this clinical strategy is associated with significant improvements in PONV outcomes for patients and staff. The results have set a new standard for PONV management in our institution.

Chapter 9

Future research strategies for prevention and treatment of PONV

Phil M Hopkins

Introduction

PONV is recognised as a most distressing complication. It ranks alongside pain as the post-operative complication most feared by patients awaiting surgery. As well as being distressing for the patient, PONV delays discharge, increases nursing workload and is costly (Sanchez *et al.* 1995). An incidence of up to 90 per cent in some surgical groups (Morris *et al.* 1998) should dictate that research into the prevention and treatment of PONV is a top priority.

There are indeed numerous reports in the anaesthetic literature of studies in the field. The area of the brain responsible for the initiation of the vomiting reflex, known as the vomiting or emetic centre, has been located to the reticular formation of the medulla (Andrews 1992). Efferent activity emanating from the vomiting centre is thought to arise in response to nociceptive afferent activity, especially that arising from abdominal and pelvic viscera. Vestibular activity is a well-known precursor of vomiting (motion sickness) as are intense emotional or psychological stimuli (Palazzo & Strunin 1984). Another region of the medulla, known as the chemoreceptor trigger zone (Borison 1989), contains a variety of receptors (Atweh & Kuhar 1977; Palacios *et al.* 1981; Wamsley *et al.* 1981; Waeber *et al.* 1988) that, when stimulated, lead to increased output from the vomiting centre. The transduction of the chemical stimulus into vomiting centre output may involve dopaminergic, cholinergic, histaminergic, serotinergic and opioid receptors, either singly or in combination. Antagonism of these receptors remains the principal pharmacological approach to the treatment and prevention of PONV (Peroutka 1982). And yet, the most successful clinical trials of any of the antagonists fail to reduce the incidence of PONV by much more than 50 per cent (see, for example, Morris *et al.* 1998). This contrasts with the situation in the prevention and treatment of cancer chemotherapy-induced nausea and vomiting, where 5-HT_3 antagonists, such as ondansetron and granisetron, have had a huge impact (Cubeddu *et al.* 1990; Kidgell *et al.* 1990; Pintens 1990). Such a difference between the two situations indicates that additional factors may be operating in PONV, as compared with chemotherapy emesis. Indeed, cohort studies and retrospective analyses have identified several factors that predispose to PONV (see, for example, Palazzo & Evans 1993). Other than specific drugs, these include female sex, age, obesity, history of motion sickness and nature of surgery (e.g. gynaecological operations). While such studies may be useful for targeting those patients at greatest risk of PONV, they give few clues as to the best approach to preventing PONV. Knowledge of these factors is also important, however, in the design of clinical trials in which as many confounding variables should be controlled as is practically feasible.

But perhaps before we discuss future clinical trials in PONV research, we should consider whether our fundamental knowledge is sufficient to dispense with further basic research. The lack of efficacy of current clinical approaches, and indeed the number of different approaches *per se*, indicate to me that we do have much to learn. In a review of limited space, such as this, it would be inappropriate to detail all the possible laboratory research angles that might be considered. Instead, I will briefly discuss three research questions that are of importance to improving the management of PONV.

Can we distinguish the properties of anaesthetic drugs responsible for the anaesthetic effect from those responsible for PONV?

The implication in asking this question is that we can identify the cellular mechanisms of anaesthesia. Importantly, however, we know that the anaesthetic properties for some groups of anaesthetic drugs do not involve mechanisms that cause nausea and vomiting. Specifically, the intravenous anaesthetics, which probably have their major anaesthetic effect through amplification of GABA-induced chloride currents (Franks & Lieb 1994), demonstrate differing propensities for inducing PONV. Thiopentone and, especially, etomidate are emetic (Horrigan *et al.* 1983; Kestin & Dorje 1987), whereas propofol is not (de Grood *et al.* 1987; Edelist *et al.* 1987), and there is some evidence that it may even have anti-emetic properties (McCollum *et al.* 1988). The situation is different with the volatile anaesthetics. These drugs also increase inhibitory chloride currents (Franks & Lieb 1994), but the magnitude of these effects is probably insufficient to explain the complete range of their anaesthetic effects. Evidence is accumulating that the volatile anaesthetics inhibit the release of excitatory neurotransmitters (Schlame & Hemmings 1995) through actions on presynaptic calcium channels and possibly also sodium channel subtypes (Lynch & Pancrazio 1994; Winlow *et al.* 1995). It can be easily envisaged how increasing inhibitory signals and inhibiting excitatory neurotransmitters might contribute to anaesthesia. It is not so clear, however, how these mechanisms would be likely to lead to increased neuronal output by the vomiting centre. Other than a potent agonistic action at some cholinergic receptor subtypes (Raines 1994), the volatile anaesthetics have little effect at receptor subtypes identified in the chemoreceptor trigger zone. This is perhaps why the conventional antagonists at these receptors appear to have limited efficacy in PONV. Many other actions of volatile anaesthetics have been described in neuronal preparations and other cell types, and some of these could plausibly lead to increased activity in the neuronal networks that make up the vomiting centre. For example, in some types of neuron, volatile anaesthetics cause an increase in intracellular Ca^{2+} concentration (Winlow *et al.* 1995), which could lead to increased neuronal activity. Such an action might, however, have a role in the anaesthetic action of these drugs. Testing of these hypotheses requires more detailed characterisation of the types of neuron present in those central pathways responsible for emetic reflexes and their responses to anaesthetic drugs.

Can the neuronal pathway of opioid-induced vomiting be identified?

Opioids are probably the single biggest culprit in causing PONV (Dundee *et al.* 1965; Pandit & Kothary 1989). The influence of opioids is perhaps more complex than might be first considered. As well as directly stimulating emesis, opioids can, through alleviation of pain, reduce nausea and the likelihood of vomiting (Anderson & Krohg 1976). The pro-emetic effects of opioids are considered to be initiated through binding to opioid (probably μ) receptors located in the chemoreceptor trigger zone. Opioid receptor antagonism is clearly not a treatment option, as the desirable analgesic effects would be antagonised also. The logical approach, therefore, would be to interrupt the pathway downstream from opioid receptor activation. Delineation of this pathway is required.

Is there a 'final common processing pathway' for the emetic reflex?

As already suggested, much more is known about the many stimuli of emesis than the neuronal pathways involved in transduction of a stimulus to produce the emetic reflex. Postulation of the vomiting centre implies that the diverse stimuli may converge to trigger a common mechanism for emesis. If this is so, the precise location of the convergence has important consequences for the likely efficacy of therapeutic interventions (Borison 1989; Andrews 1992). If we consider the vomiting centre to be a central pattern generator (CPG) – in its simplest form, a single group of identical neurons responsible for co-ordination of a defined motor response – several possibilities for afferent and efferent connections exist. Three examples are represented in Figure 9.1. The relationship in Figure 9.1(a) presents the most attractive therapeutic potential, as a drug that either reduces activity of the interneuron or blocks the effect of its neurotransmitter on the CPG should block emesis resulting from a range of stimuli. A drug that blocks the transmitter(s) released by the CPG neurons will have a similar effect. The neural connections illustrated in Figures 9.1(b) and 9.1(c) are less amenable to intervention. A drug targeted at inhibition of the CPG neurotransmitter(s) will be efficacious in the model in Figure 9.1(b) but not that in Figure 9.1(c). The connections illustrated in Figure 9.1(c) imply that multiple neurotransmitters are involved in initiation and modulation of CPG output and a combination of drugs is likely to be required to fully inhibit emesis at this level.

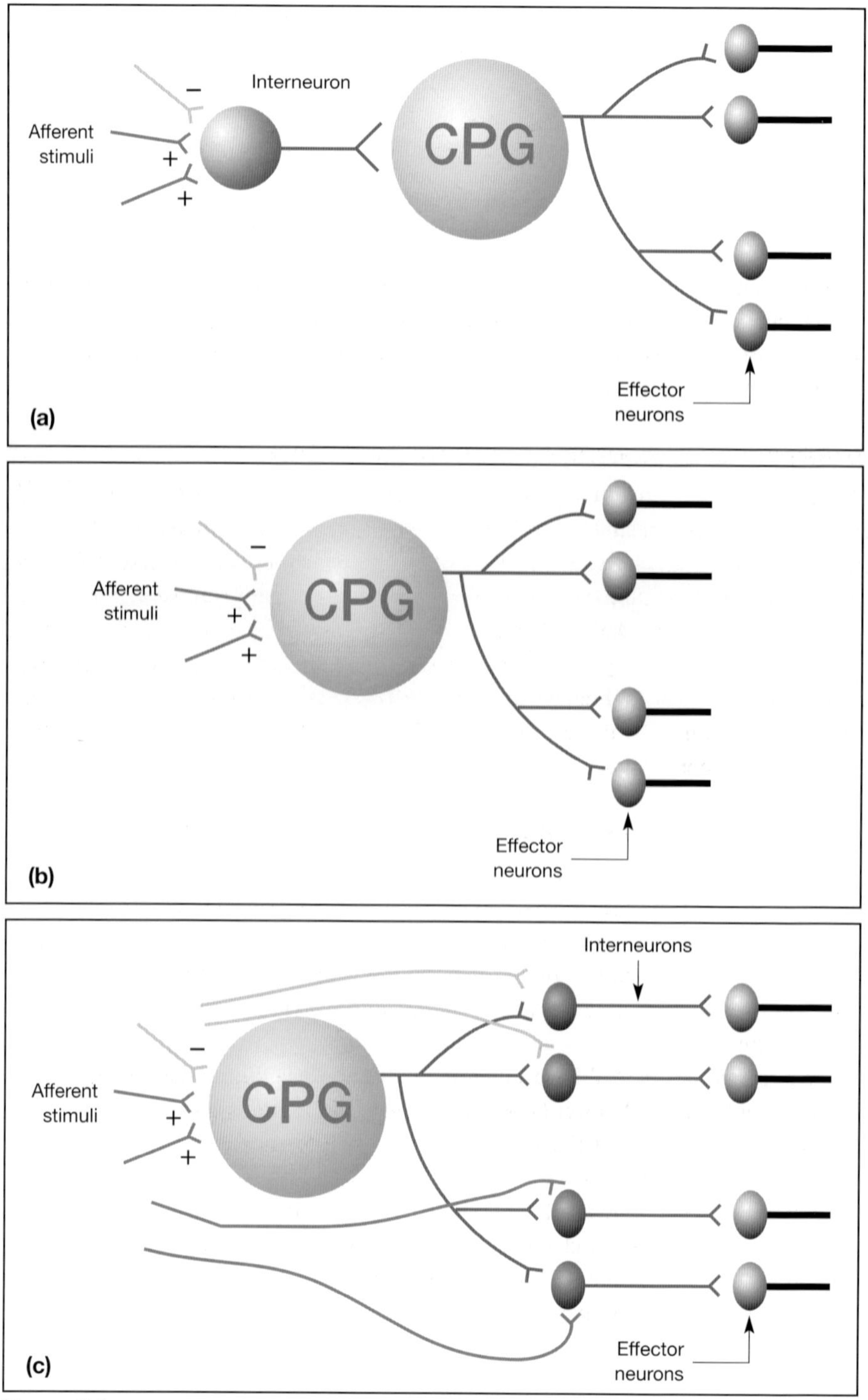
Interneuron
Afferent stimuli
−
+
+
CPG
Effector neurons
(a)
Afferent stimuli
−
+
+
CPG
Effector neurons
(b)
Interneurons
Afferent stimuli
−
+
+
CPG
Effector neurons
(c)

Figure 9.1

Recent work using CP 99,994, a substance P antagonist, suggests that the connections illustrated in Figures 9.1(a) and 9.1(b) may be good models for the CPG (Longmore *et al.* 1997). CP 99,994 has been shown in animal models to be effective against a wide range of stimuli, including cisplatin (5-HT and vagal stimulation), copper sulphate (gastric irritation), apomorphine (a dopamine [D2] receptor agonist) and morphine. Labelled antibody studies for the receptor subtype thought to be involved (neurokinin-1) would be useful to identify the location of pathways involved in the effect of CP 99,994.

A different approach to identify areas of the brain involved in the emetic response, which is applicable to humans, is the use of positron emission tomography. This imaging technique is able to display areas of increased neuronal activity and could be used, for example, to map activity in volunteers given emetogens.

Problems with laboratory research in PONV

The major problems arise with the suitability of animal models. A fundamental problem with some species, such as rats, rabbits and horses, is that they do not vomit. Dogs, cats and ferrets do vomit and are used in emesis research. However, it is not clear that the neuroanatomical connections involved in vomiting in these animals are sufficiently similar to that in humans for results to be extrapolated to humans. Animals that do vomit may respond in different ways to emetogenic stimuli compared to humans. For example, humans and dogs readily vomit when given apomorphine, whereas cats do not. It is also clearly impossible to use animals to study nausea as this is a subjective phenomenon.

Problems with PONV research in the clinical setting

Vomiting is an explicit end-point and it should be relatively easy to record the number of events. The subjectivity of nausea, however, means that comparisons between patients and especially between studies is more difficult. Verbal rating scales and visual analogue scores can be used to obtain a measure of severity of nausea, while some investigators prefer not to attempt to quantify the severity of nausea but rather record its duration.

Many studies of PONV have failed to contribute meaningful data because they lack sufficient statistical power (Watcha & White 1992). In this sense, the power of a study is the likelihood that the study will detect a difference of defined magnitude when that difference truly exists in the population. A study will lack power if too few patients or subjects are included in the sample. Determination of sample size is a key element of study design and appropriate expertise must be sought at this stage. A power calculation requires estimates of both the incidence of an event under study and the variability of any measure. A pilot study is often required to provide these estimates.

The presence of confounding variables complicates power calculations. With regard to PONV, I have already mentioned some confounding variables that have been shown to have an influence (e.g. age, sex, history of motion sickness, type of surgery, etc.) Good study design aims to limit the influence of confounding variables, first by appropriate inclusion and exclusion criteria and second by randomised allocation to treatment and control groups.

Strategies for limiting PONV

Three main approaches to limiting PONV can be defined:

- avoiding emetogenic stimuli
- prophylaxis
- treatment of established PONV.

Each of these approaches warrants further clinical research.

Reducing emetogenic stimuli

Specific triggers of PONV have been mentioned previously but there are some interesting research questions awaiting definitive study. I will deal with some illustrative cases.

The use of nitrous oxide

Several trials have investigated the influence of nitrous oxide on PONV (Lonie & Harper 1986; Korttila *et al.* 1987; Muir *et al.* 1987). The conclusions are conflicting but many of the studies are inadequately powered and do not consider confounding variables (see above). Two groups have undertaken systematic reviews in the form of meta-analyses of relevant randomised controlled trials (RCTs) (Divatia *et al.* 1996; Tramer *et al.* 1996). Both reviews were based on a similar data set, i.e. the RCTs analysed were by and large the same in both papers, but the two sets of authors drew opposite conclusions. Divatia *et al.* found that PONV was reduced when the use of nitrous oxide was avoided and recommended it not be used. Tramer *et al.*, although they found an increased risk of PONV with nitrous oxide, recommended that it should be used because in a subset of the RCTs there was an unacceptably high incidence of recall of intra-operative awareness in those patients not given nitrous oxide. This is an interesting finding, but the incidence of awareness does seem extraordinarily high. I would suggest that it is perfectly possible to ensure lack of awareness while not using nitrous oxide and would offer the possible explanation that some investigators may have subconsciously attempted to deliver less anaesthetic in order to limit PONV. The important question of the benefits or otherwise of nitrous oxide needs to be addressed in a well-designed RCT.

Choice of anaesthetic drugs

There are fairly consistent data that indicate some anaesthetics are more likely to be associated with PONV. For example, etomidate is associated with a higher incidence than thiopentone, which in turn appears to be more emetogenic than propofol (Horrigan *et al.* 1983; de Grood *et al.* 1987; Edelist 1987). It has not been defined, however, in what situations these statistical differences are likely to be clinically important. It may well be, for example, that propofol is advantageous when used as a sole anaesthetic with no, or a short-acting, opioid for surgical procedures of limited duration. But this may not be the case when the intravenous anaesthetic is used only for induction of a prolonged anaesthetic, which is followed by the use of patient-controlled analgesia with morphine. This is an example of the extent of the detail required if evidence-based clinical decision making is to improve patient care.

Optimising analgesia

There is a complex relationship between pain, analgesic drugs and PONV. The aim of management is to minimise pain, which itself is associated with nausea and vomiting (Anderson & Krohg 1976), and to limit the emetogenic effects of analgesic drugs. Much can be achieved with methods of analgesia other than systemically administered opioids as these are the main culprit for causing PONV (Dundee *et al.* 1965; Pandit & Kothari 1989). In many circumstances, opioids are the best means of treating post-operative pain and here the goals can be defined as, first, can we limit the severity of pain (e.g. by using 'pre-emptive' analgesia), and second, is there a least emetogenic method of administering opioids (e.g. by optimising patient-contolled analgesia machine settings)?

Peri-operative fluid therapy

In many countries, but not the UK, an intravenous infusion during anaesthesia is a standard of care. Small prospective studies have suggested that intra-operative fluid therapy reduces the incidence of PONV. These findings need to be verified on a larger scale. Furthermore, the optimal fluid regimen needs to be determined.

Timing of pre- and post-operative oral intake

The level of evidence here is almost at the anecdotal level. It does seem plausible to suppose that either excessive or inadequate periods of pre-operative starvation might predispose to PONV. Similarly, the timing of initial fluid and food intake post-operatively is likely to be important (van den Berg *et al.* 1987).

With each of these potential emetogenic stimuli there are other considerations for the clinician. The use of any drug or technique is associated with benefits in addition to unwanted effects. The use of nitrous oxide, discussed above, is a good example. It is important that clinical trials are designed to address wanted and unwanted effects.

Pharmacological approaches to the prevention and treatment of PONV

Although it is to be hoped that new drugs will emerge from basic research to become clinically available, there are still many unanswered questions about the use of currently available anti-emetics for the indication of PONV. Some of these questions arise because the drug was not originally licensed for this indication. Droperidol, for example, was marketed originally as a neuroleptic adjunct to anaesthesia. Some efficacy in PONV has been demonstrated, but so have side-effects which are occasionally distressing. Clinical trials to determine the optimal dose of droperidol (balancing wanted and unwanted effects) and timing of administration would be helpful. Similar studies could usefully be carried out with cyclizine and metoclopramide. The more recently introduced 5-HT_3 antagonists have been better characterised.

Specific efficacy of individual drugs

PONV is frequently considered as a single entity. There may be some benefit in attempting to identify specific triggers and, from there go on to determine the efficacy of individual drugs with respect to those specific triggers. We know that opioids, anaesthetics and visceral stimuli all cause PONV, but why should they do so by the same mechanism and, therefore, why should PONV due to each cause be equally amenable to treatment by the same drug or group of drugs? A series of carefully designed and controlled clinical trials would be needed to progress in this area.

Drug combinations

We have discussed the complex neuropharmacology of nausea and vomiting. Lack of complete efficacy of all the currently available treatments for PONV implies that either multiple receptor types, or as-yet-unidentified receptors, are involved in the production of PONV. The former hypothesis may be addressed by studying combinations of drugs that act at different receptors. If these studies are designed to include a formal evaluation of synergism, important new information about the neurophysiology of vomiting may be obtained.

Implementation of clinical research

An extensive series of RCTs would be required to address the research questions discussed above. Experimental design will be crucial. Many of the designs will require large sample sizes, and some of the study groups will have restrictive inclusion criteria. It is inevitable that adequate recruitment will demand multi-centre involvement.

Evaluation of new treatment strategies arising from research

The aim of the research described is to accumulate sufficient data to provide a detailed evidence base which will advise the formulation of treatment strategies both to prevent and treat PONV. Once designed, these treatment strategies will require prospective evaluation and audit. Included in this evaluation should be health economic analysis.

References

Anderson R & Krohg K (1976). Pain as a major cause of postoperative nausea. *Can Anaesth Soc* J **23**, 366–9.

Andrews PLR (1992). Physiology of nausea and vomiting. *Br J Anaesth* **69**(Suppl.1), 2–19.

Atweh SF & Kuhar MJ (1977). Autoradiographic localization of opiate receptors in the brain: II the brain stem. *Brain Res* **129**, 1–12.

Borison HL (1989). Area postrema: chemoreceptor circumventricular organ of the medulla oblongata. *Prog Neurobiol* **32**, 351–90.

Cubeddu LX, Hoffman IS, Fuenmayor NT & Finn AL (1990). Efficacy of ondansetron (GR 38032F) and the role of cisplatin-induced nausea and vomiting. *New Engl J Med* **322**, 810–16.

de Grood PMRM, Mitsukuri S, van Egmond J, Rutten RMJ & Crul JF (1987). Comparison of etomidate and propofol for anaesthesia in microlaryngeal surgery. *Anaesthesia* **42**, 366–72.

Divatia JV, Vaidya JS, Badwe RA & Hawaldar RW (1996). Omission of nitrous oxide during anesthesia reduces the incidence of postoperative nausea and vomiting: a meta-analysis. *Anesthesiology* **85**, 1055–62.

Dundee JW, Kirwan MK & Clarke RSJ (1965). Anaesthesia and premedication as factors in postoperative vomiting. *Acta Anaesthesiol Scand* **9**, 223–31.

Edelist G (1987). A comparison of propofol and thiopentone as induction agents in outpatient surgery. *Can J Anaesth* **34**, 110–16.

Franks NP & Lieb WR (1994). Molecular and cellular mechanisms of general anaesthesia. *Nature* **367**, 607–14.

Horrigan RW, Moyers JR, Johnson BH, Eger EI II, Margolis A & Goldsmith S (1983). Etomidate versus thiopental with and without fentanyl. A comparative study of awakening in man. *Anesthesiology* **59**, 564–9.

Kestin IG & Dorje P (1987). Anaesthesia for evacuation of retained products of conception: comparison between alfentanil plus etomidate and fentanyl plus thiopentone. *Br J Anaesth* **59**, 364–8.

Kidgell AE, Butcher ME & Brown GW (1990). Antiemetic control: 5-HT_3 antagonists. Review of clinical results, with particular emphasis on ondansetron. *Cancer Treat Rev* **17**, 311–17.

Korttila K, Hovorka J & Erkola O (1987). Nitrous oxide does not increase the incidence of nausea and vomiting after isoflurane anesthesia. *Anesth Analg* **66**, 761–5.

Longmore J, Hill RG & Hargreaves RJ (1997). Neurokinin-receptor antagonists: pharmacological tools and therapeutic drugs. *Can J Physiol Pharmacol* **75**, 612–1.

Lonie DS & Harper NJN (1986). Nitrous oxide and vomiting. The effect of nitrous oxide on the incidence of vomiting following gynaecological laparoscopy. *Anaesthesia* **141**, 703–7.

Lynch C III & Pancrazio JJ (1994). Snails, spiders and stereo specificity – is there a role for calcium channels in anesthetic mechanisms? *Anesthesiology* **81**, 1–5.

McCollum JSC, Milligan KR & Dundee JW (1988). The antiemetic effect of propofol. *Anaesthesia* **43**, 239–40.

Morris RW, Aune H, Feiss P, Hanson A, Hasselstrom L, Maltby JR, Rocke DA, Rozenberg B, Rust M & Cohen LA (1998). International, multicentre, placebo-controlled study to evaluate the effectiveness of ondansetron vs. metoclopramide in the prevention of post-operative nausea and vomiting. *Eur J Anesthesiol* **15**, 69–79.

Muir JJ, Warner MA, Offord KJ, Buck CF, Harper JV & Kunkel JE (1987). Role of nitrous oxide and other factors in nausea and vomiting. A randomized and blinded prospective study. *Anesthesiology* **66**, 513–18.

Palacios JM, Wamsley JK & Kuhar MJ (1981). The distribution of H1-receptors in the rat brain: an autoradiographic study. *Neuroscience* **6**, 15–17.

Palazzo M & Evans R (1993). Logistic regression analysis of fixed patient factors for postoperative sickness: a model for risk assessment. *Br J Anaesth* **70**, 135–40.

Palazzo MGA & Strunin L (1984). Anaesthesia and emesis: 1. Etiology. *Can Anaesth Soc J* **31**, 178–87.

Pandit SK & Kothary SP (1989). Intravenous narcotics for premedication in outpatient anaesthesia. *Acta Anaesthesiol Scand* **33**, 353–8.

Peroutka SJ & Snyder SH (1982). Antiemetics: neurotransmitter receptor binding predicts therapeutic action. *Lancet* **1**, 714–16.

Pintens H (1990). Granisetron (BRL 43694) in the treatmentof cytostatic drug-induced emesis: a summary. *Cancer Treat Rev* **17**, 307–10.

Raines DE (1996). Anesthetic and nonanesthetic halogenated volatile compounds have dissimilar activities on nicotinic acetylcholine recepto desensitization kinetics. *Anesthesiology* **84**, 663–71.

Sanchez LA, Hirsch JD, Carroll NV & Miederhoff PA (1995). Estimation of the cost of postoperative nausea and vomiting in an ambulatory surgery center. *J Res Pharm Econ* **6**, 35–44.

Schlame M & Hemmings HC Jr (1995). Inhibition by volatile anesthetics of endogenous glutamate release from synaptosomes by a presynaptic mechanism. *Anesthesiology* **82**, 1406–16.

Tramer M, Moore A & McQuay H (1996). Omitting nitrous oxide in general anaesthesia: meta-analysis of intraoperative awareness and postoperative emesis in randomized controlled trials. *Br J Anaesth* **76**, 186–93.

van den Berg AA, Lambourne A, Yazji NS, Laghari NA *et al.* (1987). Vomiting after ophthalmic surgery: effects of intraoperative antiemetics and postoperative oral fluid restriction. *Anaesthesia* **42**, 270–6.

Waeber C, Dixon K, Hoyer D & Palacios JM (1988). Localisation by autoradiography of neuronal 5-HT_3 receptors in the mouse. *Eur J Pharmacol* **151**, 351–2.

Wamsley JK, Lewis MS, Young WS III & Kuhar MJ (1981). Autoradiographic localization of muscarinic cholinergic receptors in rat brainstem. *J Neurosci* **1**, 176–91.

Watcha MF & White PF (1992). Postoperative nausea and vomiting: its etiology, treatment and prevention. *Anesthesiology* **77**, 162–84.

Winlow W, Hopkins PM, Moghadam HF, Ahmed IA & Yar T (1995). Multiple cellular and subcellular actions of general anaesthetics on cultured molluscan neurones. *Acta Biol Hung* **46**, 381–93.

Index